Praise for

MW01166813

"If you think that setting trail records is about speed and hubris, Nancy East will prove you wrong. It is not her success, but her vulnerability that will encourage you to keep moving forward when the next step feels impossible. It is not her impressive miles, but rather her insightful reflections that allow you to recognize feelings of gratitude and connectedness in the midst of pain and loss. And it is not her attributes as a hiker, but her roles as a mother, spouse, and friend that make this book a valuable resource for anyone who is trying to navigate through relationships - and adventure."

Jennifer Pharr Davis, author of *The Pursuit of Endurance: Harnessing the Record-Breaking Power of Strength and Resilience*

"Nancy P. East's account of her and Chris Ford's FKT attempt of hiking all the trails in Great Smoky Mountain National Park reveals superhuman efforts and dogged persistence. Equally impressive to the physical feat was the mental fortitude and self-examination that Nancy generously reveals in her book. It gives the reader hope that self-determination, persistence and planning can help any of us overcome obstacles and reach our goals."

Kathy Zachary, former director of Smoky Mountain Field School

"There's no disputing Nancy East's competence as an outdoorswoman. She's a member of a North Carolina search-and-rescue team that frequently responds to incidents in Great Smoky Mountains National Park.

What's also beyond dispute is East's strength as a natural storyteller, which she capably demonstrates in her book about her record-setting achievement, *Chasing the Smokies Moon*. Instead of a tedious mile-by-mile recap of her nearly month-long odyssey, East's descriptive style transports readers to the scene of the action and affords them the opportunity to experience vicariously what few people have actually accomplished and none within in a shorter timeframe.

East's 30 chapters, each of which opens with an inspirational epigraph, sustain a compelling narrative drive while gracefully interlacing memories of past adventures, reflections on life and family, and descriptions of other hikers encountered along the way. As for the latter, East has little patience for those who enter the park's backcountry ill-equipped and ill-prepared, having helped deliver a number of them—the more fortunate ones—to safety over the years."

David Brill, author of *Into the Mist: Tales of Death and Disaster, Mishaps and Misdeeds, Misfortune and Mayhem in GSMNP*

"*Chasing the Smokies Moon* is a deep dive into the depths of a Fastest Known Time record attempt. East relays with humor, profundity, and humility the highs and lows of an intense journey through the Great Smoky Mountains and human connection."

Heather Anderson, author of *Mud, Rocks, Blazes: Letting Go on the Appalachian Trail*

"This story is more than just a recounting of an incredible feat of endurance and perseverance, it is an insightful and revealing look into the mind and soul of a multifaceted, adventurous woman."

Kevin Fitzgerald, former Deputy Superintendent of Great Smoky Mountains National Park

"In this literary journey, Nancy East eloquently and transparently weaves together the narratives of her FKT attempt, fundraising efforts, and personal growth as seamlessly as the braided, blue ridges of Appalachia."

Steven Reinhold, *Backpacker Magazine*, Brand Ambassador

"An amazing feat well-planned and superbly executed. Nancy East writes from the heart about each day's challenges and joys. As exhausted as she is after hiking more than thirty miles a day, she finds the reward which makes every Smokies trail special. The reader will be with East and her hiking partner every step of the way.

Chasing the Smokies Moon might inspire some to do more hiking in the Smokies."

Danny Bernstein, author of *DuPont Forest: A History*

"Like a friend sharing stories around a campfire, Nancy East invites readers to hear the tale of the 800-mile journey taken by her and her companion in Great Smoky Mountains National Park. The Olympic-sized athletic challenge not only became an adventure in self-awareness and a test of mental and physical fortitude, but also a valuable, charitable mission. While planting record-breaking, fast-paced bootprints in Smoky Mountain history, the pair captured the gold-medal prize by surpassing the fund-raising goals to support outdoor safety programs for the public. Zip up your fleece jacket, put another log on the fire, and listen in."

Marci Spencer, author of *Clingmans Dome, Highest Mountain in the Great Smokies; Potluck, Message Delivered: "The Great Smoky Mountains are Saved!"* and books on the history of Pisgah, Nantahala and Cherokee National Forests

Chasing the
SMOKIES
MOON

**An audacious 948 mile hike—
fueled by love, loss, laughter,
and lunacy**

To Capt. Ron,
The best part of the
Smokies 900 is the journey,
so enjoy every mile, no
matter how long it takes!
Nancy East

Chasing the
SMOKIES
MOON

An audacious 948 mile hike—
fueled by love, loss, laughter,
and lunacy

NANCY EAST

Headlamp Publishing
Waynesville, NC

Edited by Steve Kemp
Cover and book design by Lisa Horstman
Cover artwork by Gay Davis Bryant
Production assistance by Elevate Interpretive Media Developers
All photos by Nancy East or Chris Ford, unless otherwise noted.

10 9 8 7 6 5 4 3 2 1

Published by Headlamp Publishing, Waynesville, NC
ISBN 979-8-9851114-0-8
Printed in U.S.A.

To Mama, my touchstone

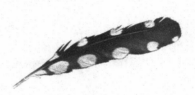

and for Larry, Aidan, Paige, and Wogene,
my heart's core

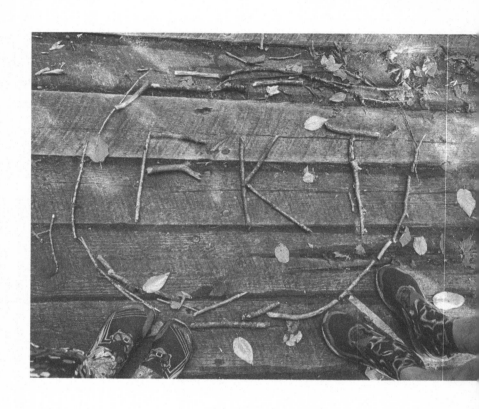

Contents

Great Smoky Mountains
National Park Trails

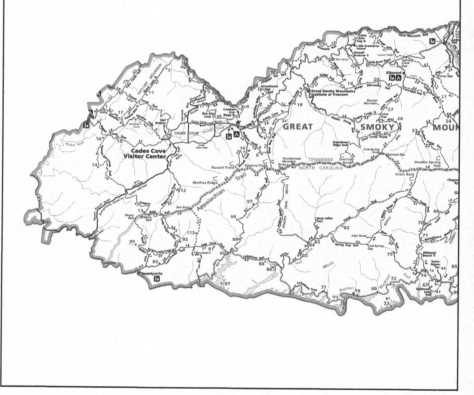

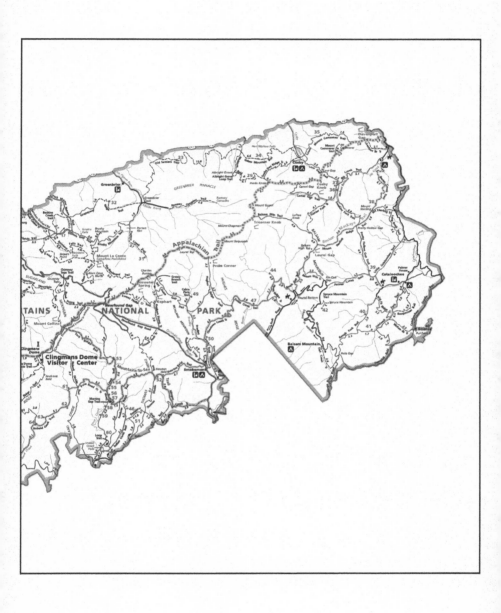

Yours is the light by which my spirit's born:
—you are my sun, my moon, and all my stars.

—EE CUMMINGS

September 30, 2018

My assigned search and rescue (SAR) team, composed of members from multiple agencies, was positioned some 600 feet below Forney Ridge Trail in the Salola Branch drainage. Even avid hikers in Great Smoky Mountains National Park had likely never heard of this creek. These rugged, off-trail areas were typically explored only by intrepid volunteers from regional SAR teams during our operations. Corey Winstead, our team's leader, instructed us to stay within line of sight of the person beside us as we descended the steep and rugged mountainside. The dense vegetation and treacherous terrain mocked Corey's commands—maintaining a straight path was impossible. The best we could do was hope to hear each other's voices or the sound of leaves crunching underfoot. But the helicopters flying closely above, also searching, made even that a challenge.

I was cautious as I descended through a patch of sizable boulders. The damp leaf litter made them as slick as oil in spots and hid the crevices between them—it would be easy to snap an ankle or a leg here. Not to mention they were the perfect habitat for timber rattlesnakes—a discovery Lane made the previous day while searching on the other side of the ridge. Luckily, the snake only gave him a stern warning, striking his hiking pole rather than his leg.

It was the fifth day of a search that would end when the body of a missing hiker was found two days later. Susan Clements, a 53-year-old woman from Ohio, was located miles from where she was last seen on Forney Ridge Trail, partially unclothed, lying in Huggins Creek.

Her autopsy determined that foul play was not involved in her death, unless you count the cruelty of Mother Nature. Susan succumbed to the end-stage effect of hypothermia, called paradoxical undressing. Victims of this phenomenon erroneously believe their body is hot rather than lethally cold. In a delusional state, they often remove clothing in an effort to cool off. Death is imminent for most at this point.

She was last seen by her college-aged daughter, Emily, whom she had hiked with that day. They were returning to the Clingmans Dome parking area after they enjoyed a three mile out-and-back day hike to Andrews Bald.

Emily ventured ahead of Susan to visit the iconic spiraling observation tower at the summit of Tennessee's tallest mountain before they left the park. They parted ways less than a mile from the parking area, on one of the most popular trails in the most visited national park in the United States.

CHAPTER ONE

Time to Set a Record

*Your feet can take you in many directions, but only your heart
can tell you what direction that is.*

—NISHAN PANWAR

September 4, 2020

My phone's alarm sounded at 10:00 p.m. I was fairly sure I had slept
for a couple of hours, but it was a brief night's rest for the energy I'd
soon expend—not to mention the odd hour to start a new day, considering the current one hadn't technically ended yet.

Excitement coupled with mild anxiety replaced my normal routine
of easing gently out of bed in a sleepy stupor. I popped up, turned on
the hotel's bedside lamp, and said aloud in a voice cloaked in doubt,
"Here we go. Time to set a record." Even after a year and a half of
training, there was still only a small part of me that believed I could
accomplish my goal. But I figured an encouraging self-pep talk, even
if it felt disingenuous, couldn't hurt.

I headed to the bathroom to start a ritual I would soon memo-
rize and repeat each morning on auto pilot: use the bathroom, put
my contacts in, brush my teeth, don my hiking dress, lubricate and
tape my feet while inspecting them for any burgeoning blisters or

1

other trouble spots, double check my food and water supply for the day, and throw my headlamp over my head—all while consuming a high calorie-laden breakfast, typically consisting of commercially packaged miniature omelettes and pancakes I reheated in the microwave, along with a banana. I didn't put my gaiters, socks, and shoes on until reaching the trailhead. Instead, I wore a comfy pair of recovery sandals. There was both a physical and mental advantage to pampering my feet every chance I had.

I stepped out of the hotel room in Cherokee, North Carolina. I was shocked to see wet pavement and light rain falling, despite the dry forecast. One should regard weather predictions in the Smokies as a loose suggestion rather than a precise verdict. Mercuriality is the nature of this temperate rainforest, which receives more rain than anywhere else in the Southeast, including Everglades National Park. Even though I knew this pattern of unpredictability well, it caught me off guard. While I still had the benefit of a roof over my head, I ensured my rain gear was readily accessible, including my umbrella in the side pocket of my backpack.

Chris Ford, one of my best friends, emerged from his hotel room a few doors down with his wife, Jamie. Chris and I had trained long and hard together just for this moment—beginning our fastest known time (FKT) attempt of hiking all 801 miles of official trail in Great Smoky Mountains National Park, a challenge referred to as the Smokies 900.

Besides her role as one of our biggest cheerleaders, Jamie graciously offered to assist us in myriad ways throughout the attempt—shuttling us to and from trailheads at unusual hours, washing our filthy laundry, having meals ready, and any other random task we might ask of her. She had more flexibility in her schedule since she was working remotely during the COVID-19 pandemic. Remote employment, however, did not diminish the workload of her demanding career. She would repeatedly rise to the occasion of helping us succeed, starting with her first day working the FKT graveyard shift.

We piled in the car to start our first of what would be many drives up U.S. Highway 441 (Newfound Gap Road), the busiest road in the park that roughly bisects it through its middle. Chris and Jamie were in good spirits, and my anxiety lessened as we ascended the mountain at an exponentially faster pace than what we would spend the next sixteen hours walking.

We turned onto Clingmans Dome Road to reach one of the highest paved trailheads in the park. Thick fog engulfed the car while the rain continued in earnest. I was concerned about Jamie driving over two hours by herself home, especially in these conditions, after dropping us off at Noland Divide Trailhead. "I wish you could text us and let us know you made it home okay," I told her, knowing we'd be deep in the park's interior with no cell service, at least until sunrise. But I suspected Chris would eventually check for a cell signal on a high ridge to confirm her return, and it put my mind at ease.

Larry, my husband, texted me and wished us luck. He also reminded me of how much he loved me, and I acutely missed his embrace while reading his message. Training and planning for this endeavor hadn't been easy on our marriage, given the time I spent consumed by it. Not to mention the time I spent working on the fundraiser our attempt supported—a preventative search and rescue program in the park to help keep visitors "safe and found" in the backcountry. Despite the challenges, Larry was my stalwart supporter, as he had been for decades.

He was at our home in Waynesville—a gateway community close to the North Carolina side of the national park—with our three sleeping kids in his charge. Leaving teenagers unattended in the middle of the night, even well-behaved ones, didn't feel like the most responsible parenting choice. But I knew all four of them were with me in spirit, despite their physical absence.

I had never been away from my family for as long as the FKT would demand. No matter how hard I tried, I couldn't shake the occasional twinge of guilt about leaving them for so long. I assuaged my self-reproach by preemptively nurturing them from afar, stocking our freezer with homemade meals and hiding love notes for each of them around our house before I left home.

Our kids were back in school, albeit remotely, and we kept extracurricular activities to a minimum to reduce exposure to the coronavirus that was wreaking havoc globally. Regardless, parenting is a demanding job. I especially wanted to make things easier for Larry since he was our primary breadwinner with a full-time career.

Shortly after receiving Larry's text, I received one from Lane Decost. Lane was one of my search and rescue teammates and a mutual friend to Chris and me. He was also our "trail boss." He had given countless hours of his time and brainpower to developing our hiking routes, revising them repeatedly to meet our requests.

As if 801 miles weren't enough, many of the trails—or segments of them—required us to hike them multiple times to connect adjoining trails. When everything was solidified, Lane had created the most efficient routes possible to hike all the official trails in Great Smoky Mountains National Park. Chris and I only needed to execute them as planned, barring any unforeseen problems like injuries or storms that created unsafe stream crossings.

I responded to Larry and Lane before placing my phone in airplane mode to preserve its battery and stuffed it into a plastic bag to protect it from the rain.

When we reached the trailhead, giddiness replaced my anxiety. I was eager to discover what my body and mind could achieve, even if it amounted to failure. Lane's words echoed in my head, "If I thought you were not up to this, I would tell you. Trust your training. Trust your body. Trust your instincts."

Chris and I both rifled through our packs to pull out our rain gear. The wind was mild, but it was enough to convince me to leave my umbrella packed away to prevent damage to it. My rain jacket and skirt were more appropriate clothing to combat hypothermia in these conditions. Ironically, the adverse conditions in which we were starting felt fitting, given the tragic event that became the catalyst for our speed record attempt.

CHAPTER TWO

Burning the Midnight Oil

I still say, 'Shoot for the moon; you just might get there!'
—BUZZ ALDRIN

September 5—39.1 miles
(5022' elevation gain, 9010' elevation loss)

When the clocks on our phones turned over to midnight, September 5, it was time to start our long walk in the Smokies. Jamie snapped a couple of photos—only our faces wearing excited smiles peeked out of our hooded rain jackets. I couldn't resist quoting a line aloud from *Talladega Nights*, one of our mutually favorite comedic movies, "If you ain't first, you're last." It did the trick to ease my last-second jitters. Over the next month, I would repeatedly discover how powerful a good sense of humor can be.

Leaving the worries of the world and its raging pandemic behind us, we began our descent down Noland Creek Trail in the fog and rain. Within the first hour of hiking, the rain tapered off and only residual drops fell from leaves of surrounding trees. The air became increasingly warm and humid as we descended into the lower elevations of the Deep Creek drainage. The sound of cicadas filled the air, amazingly loud for their diminutive size. We took a quick break to remove our rain gear when we reached the trail junction with Pole Road Creek Trail, our next leg of the route.

I walked off the trail, away from Chris to relieve my bladder. I peeked up at the sky while I squatted and noticed the nearly full moon emerging behind the shifting cloud cover. I turned off my headlamp and basked in the glow of moonlight casting lumens around me.

Back on the trail, I shared a revelation with Chris, "If we complete the FKT as planned, it will align with a complete 28-day cycle of the moon. I think today is two days removed from a full moon, so we'll hike to the light of a full one the night before we finish." This coinciding lunar cycle gave me unexpected confidence. How many moon cycles have I lived through in my forty-eight years of life, I wondered? And this effort will only take one.

The nighttime hours ticked by quickly. We passed several tents with snoring backpackers in the multiple campsites on the lower stretches of Deep Creek Trail. By the time their occupants could have donned their own headlamps to take an inquisitive peek at the strange light filling the forest nearby, we would have long slipped into the inky shadows further down the trail.

After eight hours of hiking, we turned off our headlamps to welcome the first light of day. We had descended from the highest elevations of the park to some of its lowest reaches, only to start the cycle of climbing and descending again. It's a pattern our muscles had developed a memory for, but I was still uncertain about how well mine would fare with so little rest.

A light rain fell, but it wasn't windy, so I popped my umbrella open and attached its handle to the shoulder strap on my backpack. I took a selfie with my phone and sent it to my family since I had a rare pocket of cell reception. "Morning!" is all I texted to them, knowing they were amid getting ready for work and school.

I munched on a handful of chocolate covered espresso beans while we walked the relatively easy terrain of Beaureguard Ridge along Noland Divide Trail. It sufficiently warded off my sleepiness, but Chris' weaving strides told a different story. "You're welcome to some of these espresso beans. Surprisingly, they're helping me stay awake," I said to Chris. "Nah, I'm good. I'll shake it off soon," he replied.

The previous morning, Jamie and Chris drove to Clingmans Dome to watch the sunrise; Chris was now paying the price of that early wake up call. Having the extra time with his beloved before starting this attempt was likely worth the cost of heavy eyelids. But I made a mental note to offer him my stash of espresso beans at the hotel that evening, so he'd have some during our route the following day.

Eventually, we circled to the same spot on Noland Divide Trail where we stopped many hours prior to remove our rain gear. At this 4-way junction of trails, we continued our journey to the southwest, descending Noland Creek Trail.

Shortly after leaving the trail intersection, we crossed paths with a father and son who were on their last day of a multi-day backpacking experience. They asked where we started our hike from and we told them, "Noland Divide Trail off Clingmans Dome Road. We started at midnight." We laughed after we wished them well and continued on, realizing our route and its timing must have sounded strange. They didn't know we had already hiked twenty-three miles to reach that point, rather than 3.7 miles—the distance from the trailhead at Clingman's Dome Road.

As we approached the flats of Noland Creek near campsite 62, Chris kept us entertained with a story of an encounter he had in the same area a few years prior with a female trail runner. Shortly before coming across Chris, she came across an enormous rattlesnake sunbathing across the trail. The snake was undeterred by the small rocks she picked up and threw near it, hoping it would move so she could safely pass. But the snake wasn't budging. Eventually, she turned back to retrace her steps to the trailhead, rather than continuing on her intended loop. That's when she encountered Chris, who was hiking the same loop.

Chris, well versed in venomous snake encounters in the Smokies, convinced her he'd be able to encourage the snake to move. They arrived at the spot where the runner had previously stopped. The snake lounging across the trail welcomed the two humans with an intimidating rattle from the buttons on its tail. Chris looked down and noticed another rattlesnake, even bigger than the one on the trail. Camouflaged in the underbrush, it was within easy striking distance of where the woman had been picking up rocks.

Chris' instincts took over, and he pushed the woman out of harm's way. She began screaming in fear. Chris instructed her to move into campsite 62 while he continued to problem solve this potentially dangerous situation. He eventually used his hiking pole to pick up the snake on the trail and move it. The snake's weight was so great it bent his pole in a wide arc, and the snake in the brush began rattling in protest against his comrade's relocation.

"The noise from both snakes rattling together bounced around in a stereo effect, and it sounded like there were more than two of them there," Chris explained to me. Luckily, there were just two. Snakes and humans all survived the encounter unscathed, but the lone hiker wasn't about to leave Chris' side until they emerged safely onto Clingmans Dome Road!

The rest of our day was not nearly as eventful, though Chris' hazy, sleep-deprived state resolved as he retold his adrenaline-filled, "Tale of Two Serpents."

After a nearly 6-mile out-and-back leg on Springhouse Branch Trail, we polished off the route with a final descent down Noland Creek Trail—an unpaved roadbed, open only to pedestrians and horses. It was encouraging to end our day at a quicker pace. We reached my waiting car at 2:30 p.m., which we had shuttled to this location the evening prior.

We made the drive back to our hotel in Cherokee where we made hasty phone calls to our families, consumed massive quantities of pizza, and scurried to reset our gear for our second day of hiking, which would begin in a few hours.

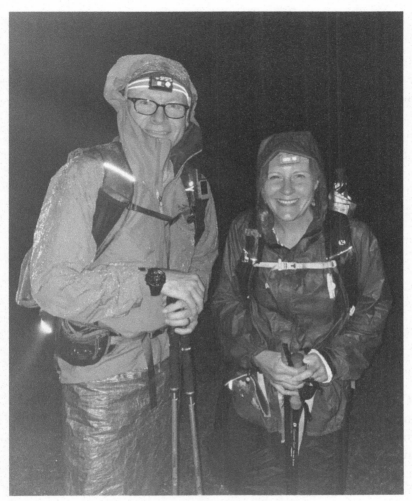

DAY 1: Chris and Nancy just before the clock started.

CHAPTER THREE

The New Normal

You never really understand a person until you consider things from his
point of view... until you climb into his skin and walk around in it.

—ATTICUS FINCH, *TO KILL A MOCKINGBIRD*

Day 2—36.2 miles
(5,886' gain, 9,504' loss)

Our second day began much like the first, descending from Clingmans Dome Road, but without rain and a start time of 2:00 a.m.
rather than midnight. It was also slightly cooler, and the chill in the
night air helped keep me alert. This was fortuitous because I needed to stay attentive on Fork Ridge Trail's uneven, rocky terrain and
narrow, off camber sections that mandated careful foot placement.

Chris was swifter and more sure-footed on the descent, but he was
patient with my slower pace. We discovered salamanders frequently
on the rocks we walked on, and one of them leapt into the night air as
Chris' foot barely missed it. I wondered what the salamanders thought
of the enormous creatures wandering the wilderness at night with a
bright cyclops eye blinding them.

Five miles in, we reached Deep Creek. I acknowledged the impossibility of keeping my feet dry while I crossed. I waded through in

10

my trail runners without an ounce of regret—I knew my feet would eventually get wet on deeper crossings later that morning. Chris was gifted with long legs and inherent bravery which gave him confidence to leap between widely spaced boulders and stick each landing. This was a routine occurrence on water crossings—Chris getting to the other side with dry feet. Me, not so much.

Taking good care of our feet was a top priority during the FKT. After all, we were asking them to walk an average of 64,000 steps daily while keeping their complaints to a minimum. Things like sustained exposure to water, heat (or cold) and constant friction were their enemies. Preventative care *off* the trail was the key to keeping them happy *on* the trail: trimming our toenails, applying various specialty lotions to soften our skin, sanding calluses off with motorized foot files, and even taping sensitive areas of our feet and toes with Leukotape, a medical tape created for physical therapists but used commonly in the hiking world to ward off blisters.

Hikers often erroneously view calluses as a coat of armor for feet, toughening them for the rigors of the trail. In reality, calluses are problems. Our odd but pragmatic goal was to make our feet as smooth as a baby's bottom. All it took was one blister forming under a thick callus on my heel for me to understand this rationale—it was nearly impossible to treat and caused constant pain. If we stood a chance of enduring the abuse we'd put our feet through during the FKT, Chris and I needed to be hypervigilant about pampering them.

After the water crossing, we climbed Deep Creek Trail to its start on Newfound Gap Road, only to turn around and repeat the same 3.9 miles downhill. Eventually, our feet hit a new stretch of the same trail, and we continued on through what we dubbed Jurassic Park of the Smokies.

Deep Creek Trail is fourteen miles long, and its middle section, especially, has a primordial feel. In some places, the dense vegetation completely covered the trail. In other areas, there was extensive damage from flash floods, obliterating parts of the trail and causing short but time-consuming workarounds. Numerous blowdowns were also strewn across the trail at frequent intervals. Some had fallen in a way that required us to play a hiker's version of Twister through the dense branches. Despite the tree limbs clawing at our own limbs as we climbed up, over, under, and through them, we laughed at the absurdity of our effort.

We reached the junction with Martins Gap Trail and began the next phase of our day, which entailed a deliberate pattern of weaving on and off multiple trails in the Deep Creek network. A popular area with the local community, the well-groomed trails allowed us to rack up miles at a faster pace. We checked and double checked our map, so as not to strand a straggler section of trail. Nothing would have been more discouraging and threatening to our success, so Chris was careful to reference our map frequently, both on and off trail.

As we hiked along, I reminisced about an unexpected search and rescue effort I handled during a solo hike the previous January. I was hiking down Indian Creek Motor Trail on a cold rainy morning, the temperature barely cresting 40 degrees, when I noticed two teenage boys running toward me from the opposite direction. "Hey, do you know where you are?" they yelled as I approached them. They were both shivering in their drenched cotton clothing. "Yeah, I know exactly where I am, but it looks like you're not so sure," I replied.

"We were running ahead of our school group to get to a waterfall, but we couldn't find it. Then we tried to make a loop back to the van, but we're lost. We wondered if we might see cars on this trail because of its name," they told me.

They were miles away from where they started at the Deep Creek trailhead. I needed to think fast. Standing idle in the steady rain would only worsen their mildly hypothermic state. It was a matter of time before they transitioned from only shivering to a state of the "umbles,"—mumbles, fumbles, and stumbles—all symptoms of a person's core body temperature sliding into a potentially lethal zone.

They didn't hesitate when I asked them to remove their shirts while I dug in my backpack for dry clothing for them to wear. Next, I handed one of them my umbrella so they stood a better chance of staying dry in my synthetic and merino wool clothing. They also didn't flinch at donning a bright pink rain jacket and woman's shirt, but they needed help to put them on since their hands had lost some motor control.

"You guys need to trust that I can get you out of here and follow me as quickly as your legs will let you," I said firmly. I knew they were physically exhausted, but they needed to keep moving. Otherwise, I'd need to set up the lightweight tarp I carried with me on my hikes—in case I needed an emergency shelter—and start a fire to warm them back up. But that would be a far more complicated and time-consuming solution in the pouring rain.

Without complaint, we started hiking. As we walked, one of them confessed, "Just before we saw you, we were about to head up the hill off the trail. We thought we might be able to see better." This news was alarming. Once a lost person leaves a trail, they become a proverbial needle in a haystack and the odds of a search and rescue team finding them, if ever, decreases with each passing hour.

"But then we saw you in the distance and you had hiking sticks. We figured you probably knew what you were doing if you had those." I was amused by their comment, but until we arrived at my car several miles away, it was hard to laugh at anything.

The story ended well. We were lucky because I eventually caught a cell signal. I called the park's dispatch number to discover that the school mentors had reported the boys missing. We made our way back to my waiting car at Thomas Divide trailhead. The boys ended up hiking fourteen miles instead of their intended 3-mile route. I drove them down to Deep Creek Trailhead, where the rest of their group finally emerged from the trail.

The mentors and the other students were soaking wet, depleted of physical and emotional energy—none of them were dressed any better than the boys. Once they assured me they could drive the school van safely, I bid them farewell and wished them well. I hoped they had all learned a valuable lesson or two that day.

Afterward, I couldn't stop thinking about what might have happened if I hadn't come across them. Did the mentors even realize the danger they put their students and themselves in? Would they know how to make better choices before the next hike? The only thing that made sense was contacting the school's director to relay the story. He assured me he would take steps to provide training for his staff before allowing them to lead hikes again.

A year and a half later, I would learn that the school closed after multiple incidents of purported student neglect, cited in a 158-page state-issued report. Staff not having proper training or support to lead students into backcountry settings was a common theme. The report included the day I came across the boys in the woods, stating that the school had never notified the parents of what happened. One of the boys I helped was quoted: "It was pretty scary—we ran into a woman who worked for the forest department and she had extra clothes and food and we warmed up in her car." Irrespective of him thinking I worked for "the forest department," (those "hiking sticks" really made an impression), I was thankful he understood the gravity of the situation, even if I felt the school never did. A nonchalant social media post with a picture from the hike, the caption reading, "Boys did rain hike to test their endurance," was all I needed to prove my theory.

My thoughts drifted back to the present. Chris and I ended the day with a waiting car at the same trailhead where I had emerged with the boys back in January. We had positioned the car two days prior in anticipation of needing it at the end of our route. But now, I was hiking expeditiously out of the woods for an altogether different reason; ironically, for a cause whose goal was to prevent future incidents like the one I found myself in that cold, dreary day. The second day of the attempt behind us, we drove back to Cherokee for another brief night's sleep.

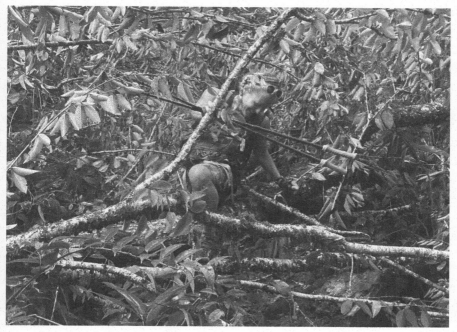

DAY 2: On Deep Creek Trail.

CHAPTER FOUR

In the Beginning

I am always more interested in what I am about to do
than what I have already done.

—RACHEL CARSON

Day 3—35.8 miles
(8011' gain, 9572' loss)

Mount Le Conte, one of the most iconic and recognizable peaks in the Smokies, patiently awaited our return after countless miles of training on its flanks. Once again, we started hiking in the dark with Orion the Hunter standing guard over us in the night sky. Each day, for the first five days of our attempt, we slid the clock forward two more hours before we started hiking. This allowed us to start our ascent of Alum Cave Trail at a slightly more reasonable time of 4:00 a.m. The reward of catching the sunrise on Le Conte's summit in return for a 5-mile hike attracted other hikers as well. It was one of the few routes where we knew we'd have company at such an early hour.

The smell of sulfur wafted through the air as we approached Alum Cave. We didn't pass the usual throngs of crowds congregating under and around the overhanging bluff. It was still too early for that, at least.

Chris took my photo as I walked through the mineral-rich, dusty soil, my headlamp shining brightly against its wall and the condensation from my breath visible in the chilly morning air.

By the time we reached the 6,593-foot summit of Le Conte, the first light of day was peeking over the horizon with a spectacular array of pinks and oranges hugging the silhouette of distant mountains. We made quick work of our descent down the Boulevard Trail as the sky continued to lighten and the sun rose to salute the new day. As soon as we hit the Appalachian Trail, our solitude ended as we encountered dozens of hikers heading towards Charlies Bunion, another popular destination in the park.

Many of the hikers we passed were wearing cotton clothing, inappropriate footwear, and some didn't even have water with them. I wondered how many of them were prepared to spend hours in the woods if they tripped over an exposed root or slipped off a wet boulder and injured themselves.

I suspected that none of them knew orthopedic injuries are the most common cause of rescues in the park. It would take hours for a SAR team to come to their aid and bring them to safety, even just a few miles from a trailhead. Were they prepared if it started raining? Did they have enough layers to keep their bodies warm in the cool night air?

At the junction of the Appalachian and Sweat Heifer trails, we encountered a trio of young adult men whose appropriate gear and hiking clothing set them apart from most of the other hikers we passed. One of them made eye contact with me and looked surprised. "Are you Nancy?" he asked. "Yes, but how in the world did you know that?" I replied. "I recognize you from Instagram. You guys are going after the FKT, right? I've been following you."

This exchange flattered and humbled me. Clark Newsom, an athletic trainer, and his brothers, were young enough to be my sons. Yet throughout our brief conversation, I sensed he believed in my middle-aged strength to achieve this ambitious feat of endurance.

In my mind's eye, I was still a 20-something-year-old just getting started in life. But mirrors are like that friend who keeps it real and tells you the truth. My grandmother's grey-blue eyes stared back at me now, reminding me of how she looked when I was a little girl staring into hers. No matter how young at heart I remained, Father Time was always molding me into a more aged version of myself.

I once thought my parents were past their prime when they turned forty, despite their youthful genes and active lifestyles telling a completely different story. It was the narrative our culture had instilled in me though, given the jovial antics that usually accompanied the milestone birthday. And here I was, nearly a decade beyond that. Old age is the only prejudice we outgrow, but Clark seemed immune from the common bias. We would encounter many hikers following our attempt throughout the course of our hike, but this exchange with an unlikely young follower reminded me to look at myself with a more discerning eye.

It also reminded me of how far I'd come since talking about attempting the FKT on a backpacking trip in the Smokies a year and a half prior. Chris and Lane both joined me for a week long adventure on the Benton MacKaye Trail, along with Sharon McCarthy, a friend whose acquaintance I initially made online through our hiking blogs.

Chris and I were hiking along Mount Sterling Ridge Trail, with Lane and Sharon a short distance behind us. As is typical between friends on hikes, we quickly bypassed small talk for more meaningful conversation, and I shared my dream of attempting the Smokies 900 FKT with him.

The Smokies 900 is a popular challenge with hikers in Great Smoky Mountains National Park. It entails hiking all 801 miles of trails on the $1 map available in visitor centers and kiosks around the park. Around 600 people had added their name to the roster by that point. It was debatable how "900" ended up in the name, but most people thought it stemmed from the park once having over 900 miles of trails before some of them were decommissioned for various reasons.

Chris was hiking ahead of me, and I was glad he couldn't see the shocked look on my face when he disclosed he was thinking about pursuing the same thing. Or when my jaw dropped when he shared his intention to complete the challenge in thirty days or fewer. Chris' face likely had a similar look of shock. Until then, he had only told Jamie and Lane about his idea. And until that moment, Larry and Lane were my only confidantes.

A retired United States Air Force veteran, Chris had completed the Smokies 900 Challenge once and was close to finishing it again, had hiked the entire Appalachian Trail, and he was hiking the Pacific Crest Trail that summer. He wanted to attempt the FKT in the fall when he returned home from his long walk out west. I knew Chris wouldn't share this goal with me if he didn't intend on attempting it. I also knew he had the hiking chops to achieve it. Plus, he had something in his favor that I lacked—spousal support for an FKT attempt.

Before I left for our backpacking trip, I tested the waters of my FKT idea with Larry, who dismissed it. He quickly reminded me of how difficult it would be to tend to our three children by himself for nearly six weeks, even if I returned home most evenings with my 40-day plan (the record at the time was forty-three days, held by Benny Braden, a hiker from East Tennessee).

My mother once gave me an anthology of essays and quotes as a birthday gift. Of all the book's inspirational content, she told me that one particular quote by Vincent Van Gogh reminded her of me more than any other: "In spite of everything, yes, let's!" My mom knew me better than anyone. But after thirty-five years of knowing each other, Larry did, too. He was well versed in outlandish ideas I brought to him for spousal support.

Larry's career afforded him a flexible schedule, but his salary was our primary source of income. Since I only worked a limited part-time schedule as a veterinarian, my primary role was to do the heavy lifting to meet the needs of our kids and to keep our household running smoothly. But it was just a few more months before Aidan, our oldest child, would be driving. I planned to revisit the idea with Larry once Aidan could help shuttle our other two kids to and from school and their extracurricular activities.

Now, here on the trail with Chris, I felt even more deflated than when Larry brought me back to earth. Chris could crush the current record, and I only wanted to beat it by a few days. I had never hiked a long trail like Chris had, so I didn't know how well my body would—or more importantly, wouldn't—hold up during an FKT attempt spanning nearly 1,000 miles. Besting the current record by a day or so felt within the realm of possibility, given my non-existent long-distance hiking history. But thirty days or fewer? Far into the outer limits of impossibility.

Attempting to lessen the awkwardness of two friends sharing a goal that would put them in competition with each other, I told Chris I'd be his number one fan and supporter when he attempted the FKT. My words were sincere, but they carried an undertone of disappointment that I hoped he wouldn't detect.

Despite my disheartening conversations with Larry and Chris, I still couldn't let go of the idea. Attempting a speed record arose from a desire to scratch an itch of middle-aged awareness. I wanted to do something big athletically before I was too old to withstand the demands on my body (never mind that I'd never excelled in athletic endeavors at any point in my life). But the thoughts had evolved into something much bigger. I laid awake in my tent that night, reflecting on a time one month prior—the night when the idea of attempting the speed record became less about me and more about others.

I received a message on my phone while I was rinsing dinner dishes to load into the dishwasher. The message came from an acquaintance who followed my blog and knew about my involvement in the search for Susan Clements. She shared a link to a series of YouTube videos that Elizabeth Clements, Susan's youngest daughter, created during the week SAR teams searched for her mom.

I dried my hands so I could click on the link which started the first video, and I finally tore myself away from my phone's screen when I heard the dishwasher cycle finishing up several hours later. I sat entranced, watching Elizabeth's vulnerability and raw emotion.

Elizabeth was about to go to sleep in her home in Cincinnati when she received a text from Emily, her sister, that read, "Mom is missing on the trail. Park rangers are looking for her." Elizabeth was expecting a phone call or text from her mom and sister that evening. She knew they had gone on a hike together that day while passing through the Smokies on a road trip, but this was not what she was expecting to hear. "This is when my whole life changed," she explained to her audience in her first YouTube video, while blinking back tears.

Each day Susan's close-knit family held onto the thread of hope that we'd find her alive. "The whole week we were there seems like one drawn out long nightmare," Elizabeth confessed. It was heart wrenching to witness someone as young as her losing her mother to something preventable, had she known some basic safety measures to follow on a hike.

"Things like this should never happen," I said aloud. I knew the park wanted to implement a robust preventative search and rescue (PSAR) program, but as was often the case with the most visited national park that didn't even require an entrance fee, the funding wasn't there. Friends of the Smokies, a local nonprofit organization, often took on the heavy lifting of fundraising for the park's needs. There was a line item in their 2019 budget to raise funding for the PSAR program.

We all have causes that strike chords within our hearts, and this was one that began beating against mine loudly. After watching the videos, I could no longer ignore the park's need for funding. I had to figure out a way to raise the money for them.

Over the next week, I pondered various ideas and remembered how much attention the Smokies 900 FKT had received when Braden set the record. I wondered if an average hiker attempting the FKT, whose strength might be underestimated, would grab the attention of the Smokies community. If it did, would I be able to raise the money while also injecting hiker safety and preparedness tips during my hike through pre-scheduled social media posts? Surely being on a search and rescue team would give me some credibility on the topic, I thought.

The park needed $40,000 to implement the PSAR program. I figured with proper training I might stretch myself far enough athletically to achieve the FKT in forty days, and I came up with a catchy name for the fundraiser—"40K in 40 Days." It was all but settled in my mind. I just needed to convince Larry that it was a great idea, too.

The next morning on our backpacking trip, I enthusiastically said to Chris, "You know, if you wanted to wait until next spring, we could attempt the FKT together!" Desperate to hang onto my dream, the idea felt logical the night before when I came up with it in my tent. But now the words sounded ridiculous as they spilled from my mouth, and I immediately regretted saying them.

Despite Chris and I getting along very well and our hiking styles and speeds aligning nearly perfectly, I expected him to decline. Chris might not want to share the title, especially since it would mean conceding to a less competitive effort. I suspected he was trying to be polite and not hurt my feelings when he said little about my idea.

"It's for the best. You'd probably just fail anyway, even if you only tried to beat the record by one day," I thought to myself sullenly. How quickly I reverted to self-deprecation and doubt—a pattern I'd mastered over my forty-seven years. It was the comfort zone of my confidence—feigning indifference while validating my weaknesses.

Another day of our backpacking trip passed before Chris disclosed he had been pondering my idea. It surprised no one more than me when he said he liked the concept of attaching the FKT effort to a cause. He also liked the idea of attempting it together. I was shocked but excited about the possibility.

Lane, who overheard this conversation, was undoubtedly contemplating his potential role in the endeavor—logistics and route planning, something at which he excelled. Eventually, he would take on the enormous feat of unwinding the Gordian Knot of Smokies trails.

It didn't take long for my excitement to be replaced with fear, however. Did this mean Chris would swallow his pride and hike shorter days in the name of a good cause? Or was he assuming I would train and feel more confident in my abilities to achieve a sub 30-day record, all while raising a young family and trying to maintain some small semblance of my career as a veterinarian? But first things first—what would our spouses think of this plan?

Larry had met Chris briefly, but I had never met Jamie. What would she think about her husband spending nearly a month in the woods with another woman? I knew my intentions were pure, but I couldn't fault Jamie if she was skeptical and mistrusting of them without knowing me. Even with all the obstacles that lay ahead, I couldn't help but wonder if we could pull this thing off together, all while raising much needed funds for the park.

The weariness in my leg muscles snapped my attention and focus back to the present. Chris may have eventually convinced me I was capable of a more ambitious FKT, but this day's route was whispering to me otherwise. As if hiking nearly thirty-six miles wasn't enough, it also held the most elevation gain *and* loss of all our routes—over 8,000 feet of ascent and 9,572 feet of descent. "C'mon legs, you've done something harder than this route, on some of these same trails, too," I told myself, attempting to shift my attention to something other than my fatigue.

The previous October, Chris and I had completed the Tour de Le Conte, a 45-mile route that entails hiking to the iconic summit three times and returning to its base accordingly. With roughly 11,000 feet of elevation gain and the same amount of loss, the route incorporates all five trails leading to Mount Le Conte's summit. The unofficial time limit for completing the challenge is twenty-four hours. Chris and I achieved it in sixteen hours, thirteen minutes, earning us a mixed-gender FKT on the route.

By then, both of our spouses had given us their blessing to partner up for the Smokies FKT fundraiser, and Friends of the Smokies welcomed our help to raise money for the PSAR program. Our Tour de Le Conte hike was a proving ground—to see how well we worked as a team under tension, how well our bodies would hold up to the rigors of high mileage training, and how successfully we could execute a fundraiser with an attention-grabbing FKT attempt. We succeeded on all three counts. The 2-year restoration project of Trillium Gap Trail, one of the trails leading to Mount Le Conte's summit, benefitted from the $7,000 that we raised for it.

While speed is the name of the game in any FKT attempt, our pace during the Smokies 900 Miler FKT would need to be significantly slower in order to achieve success. "Slow down to go faster," Chris reminded me frequently during our training hikes. With the experience of two long distance thru hikes, Chris' body had a remarkable memory for the balance between speed and risk of injury.

Reminiscing about our Tour de Le Conte effectively distracted me from the rigor of the day. By the time we reached Dry Sluice Gap Trail and started our knee-jarring descent, I focused on the abundance of gifts the trail laid out before me—late blooming wildflowers of summer, glimpses of fall in the surrounding tree color, and the multitude of various mushroom species we passed.

"One of my biggest goals is to never lose sight of how special it is to hike in this park every day. I hope I don't lose my sense of wonder out here," I said to Chris. He agreed with this sentiment, but his history of long distance hiking was a more reliable indicator of how he'd feel by the end. Despite my concern, the landscape continued to impress, with everything from epic vistas to the treasures of the forest floor, including a curious garter snake and the tiniest of toads we came across shortly after the conversation.

While filtering our water at the Cabin Flats backcountry campsite, we couldn't resist removing our shoes and socks so we could soak our feet in the cold, refreshing water of Bradley Fork Creek. My ability to keep my feet submerged indefinitely astounded Chris. The numbing effect of the water was the greatest gift of the day, and it was far more bearable than the hot, throbbing pain I experienced during our descent. I savored every moment of the experience, sitting beside one of the most idyllic creeks in the Smokies.

The soothing effect of creek water on my feet didn't last long. By the time we were descending steep, rocky Bradley Fork Trail a couple of hours later, my feet again took center stage. To add to my discomfort, I was noticing an increasingly bothersome ache in my knees. An encounter with a father and his teenage daughter provided an interesting distraction. The pair was heading towards campsite 47 for the night and asked us for navigational help.

Instead of carrying a paper map, the father had downloaded the Guthook app for the Benton MacKaye Trail, relying on it as his sole navigational tool. It was obvious he didn't understand how to use it or that their planned route eventually moved off the Benton MacKaye Trail and onto other trails. Chris gave him a quick tutorial. It relieved him to hear that he didn't have to climb 5,000 more feet as he had thought—at most, they were facing 500 feet of elevation gain.

I felt a renewed sense of conviction in our goal to raise funds for a robust PSAR program in the park after passing countless ill-prepared hikers on the Appalachian Trail and in this interaction. We routinely came across hikers relying only on technological devices for navigation. Aside from the risk of phones and GPS units breaking or losing their charge, many hikers didn't even know how to use them properly for navigation, much less a map and compass.

We ended the day on a high note with some trail magic. Lane and our mutual friend, Helen Mary Cowart, prearranged to meet us in front of the Oconaluftee Visitor Center. Helen Mary brought us homemade brownies, and we ate them while plopped down on the pavement, giving our feet every second of rest we could squeeze in. The sweetest treat, however, was enjoying a quick but uplifting conversation with two friends before scrambling towards bed once again.

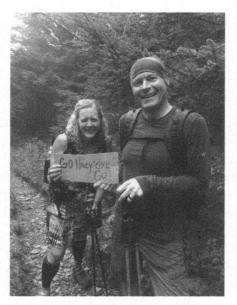

DAY 3: Nancy and Chris at Mount Le Conte's summit during the Tour de Le Conte FKT.

CHAPTER FIVE

Thumbs Down

Nature's first green is gold, Her hardest hue to hold.
—ROBERT FROST, *NOTHING GOLD CAN STAY*

Day 4—35.8 miles
(7674' gain, 7731' loss)

"Should we be going downhill?" I asked. Having started Newton Bald Trail a few minutes prior in the darkness of early morning, something didn't feel right. A quick glance at Gaia, the navigational app we used on our phones, revealed that we had mistakenly veered onto a horse trail instead of sticking to the main trail. We back-tracked, thankful we discovered the snafu quickly but annoyed at ourselves for adding a half mile to an already long day.

The physical exertion required to climb Newton Bald replaced our frustration in short order as we huffed and puffed up it. The rising sun over the horizon rewarded us, casting a brilliant amber glow onto the mountainside. Bathed in golden light, I closed my eyes for a moment and whispered a silent prayer of gratitude. Witnessing the perpetual cycle of energy manifest in the first light of day spoke to my soul more than any religious text ever had.

Two of the most recognized transcendentalists—Ralph Waldo

Emerson and Henry David Thoreau—wrote at length of finding God in nature, believing the natural world was the closest humans could come to a divine power. Emerson's words, "All I have seen teaches me to trust the creator for all I have not seen," aligned perfectly with my beliefs. But some of the former inhabitants of the lands on which we were walking, native Cherokee, were my greatest models for reverence. To the Cherokee, there wasn't a separation from physical and spiritual realms. They formed deep relationships with elements of the natural world through daily interaction and rituals. Nowadays, people are more likely to associate all the things that sustain them with man-made inventions rather than the natural world. As evidence, ask a child (or most adults) where their water comes from. The majority will say a faucet in their home rather than a river.

The closest I'd come to understanding the Cherokee way of life was attending classes hosted by a close family friend, Mark Warren, at his camp in Dahlonega, Georgia—Medicine Bow. What I learned from Mark enriched my time in the backcountry more than any of the lightweight gear I owned ever could. Creating fire from friction, using native plants medicinally or for food, as well as stalking and tracking wild animals were skills I seldom used on hikes but valued knowing. The most important thing I learned, however, is that deep in my DNA remains an atavistic yearning for communing with the earth and a higher power conjointly.

The morning passed, and the day warmed up as we descended Newton Bald. On our ascent back up Newton Bald on the Deeplow Gap Trail, we noticed an abundance of dog tracks in the area. We suspected they belonged to hound dogs, brought in by bear hunters who accessed the park in this fairly remote region. I was shocked, not because of the illegal activity of the hunters, but from a realization I had when finding these tracks. I may not have possessed the sensitive intuition of the Cherokee, but I had enough knowledge in my head to help solve a lingering mystery.

After hiking this same route together a couple of months prior, Chris texted me a photo of his ankle with an angry track of inflammation running along it. The red line wove up his ankle like the winding curves of a mountain road, faintly reminding me of poison ivy rashes Larry suffered from occasionally.

But there was one hitch—exposure to poison ivy never bothered Chris. And it looked like something was literally crawling under the surface of his skin, burrowing further up his leg each day. Turns out, that's exactly what was happening. A trip to the doctor revealed he had acquired a zoonotic (a disease that has jumped from an animal to humans) case of hookworms called cutaneous larval migrans, most likely from mud that splashed up onto his ankle, giving the hook-worm larvae an easy entry point to parasitize their next host.

Chris thought Towstring Trail, an often-muddy trail used by horse concessioners in the park, was the original source of his infestation. My veterinary mind eliminated that theory, as horses aren't susceptible to hookworm infestations. Dogs, however—especially hunting dogs who sadly don't always receive veterinary care such as deworming—are prime culprits for dropping feces laden with hookworm eggs.

Chris was successfully treated for hookworms before our FKT attempt started, but it took two doses of deworming to get the job done. Meanwhile, Jamie went to great lengths to rid his socks and gaiters of any potential parasites, too—washing them repeatedly in boiling water, then disinfecting them with multiple concoctions she deemed worthy of killing any living creature that could still be taking up residence in the fibers. I half expected to hear she subjected Chris to the same treatments before allowing him back in their bed!

I wasn't as fortunate tying up the loose ends of previous hiking-re-lated mishaps, however. The last miles of our day were my most taxing thus far because of my lingering issue. My left hand was throbbing from a surgery I had undergone twelve days prior. I was doing my best to maintain a positive mental attitude, something I preached regularly to hikers when faced with an uncomfortable situation in the backcountry.

But the custom splint I was wearing every minute of the day, unless I was showering, was hot and uncomfortable. And my salty sweat seeping into the incision line contributed to my discomfort. Despite the pain, even though my sullen attitude didn't reflect it, I was grateful to be on the other side of surgery before our FKT began.

August 7, 2020

"Damn it, that really hurt!" I yelled. Chris pivoted quickly, his eyes wide in surprise as he watched me pick myself up off one of the easiest stretches of the Appalachian Trail through the park. I had fallen forward onto my hands and knees while walking over a patch of grass, slick from morning dew. I rarely fell while hiking, and I had never sustained an injury from a fall other than a bruised ego.

"Are you ok?" Chris asked.

"I'm not sure. My hand hurts like hell. I think I fell directly on my left thumb and hyperextended it."

"Wow, yeah, I'll bet that's painful. You probably jammed it pretty good. I completely understand if you want to cut the hike short and call it a day."

We were nine miles into a 36-mile day hike, one of our last big training hikes before starting our FKT attempt in three weeks. "No, I'm good, let's keep going. It's just pain and I can work through it. I wish I could move my thumb though—it's completely locked up."

As the day wore on, I questioned my sanity for continuing, especially on Gunter Fork Trail which was one of the most rugged and physically demanding trails in the park. My hand became increasingly bruised and swollen, and I foolishly hiked in constant burning pain, not even taking the time to dig through my pack to retrieve my first aid kit with ibuprofen in it. "Today is a test of your strength and you need to see what you can endure," I thought to myself. "If you complain too much, Chris is going to question your ability to get through the FKT without falling apart."

Nothing could be further from the truth, and I knew it. Chris and I had hiked thousands of miles together in the last year and a half, pushing our bodies further and further through discomfort. Even so, I never wanted to be an emotional burden to my friend who had always consistently believed in my abilities far more than I believed in them myself.

Three days later, my hand was no better. It was still swollen, and I couldn't bend my thumb or oppose it to my pinky finger. I begrudgingly visited a walk-in clinic at a local orthopedic doctor's office. "You have a complete tear of your ulnar collateral ligament and an avulsion fracture, too. It's commonly referred to as gamekeeper or skier's thumb, and it's why you've lost the ability to oppose your thumb. The only way to repair it is with surgery," the doctor told me matter-of-factly.

"If you delay it, it will become a much more involved surgery and reconstruction with cadaver tissue will be necessary," he explained. "But your timeline is too tight to have the surgery before your hike—you can't have it done and then go do something that extreme." I left his office discouraged but not defeated. Surgery would still have to wait.

A week later, I sat in the office of Dr. Doug Gates, the hand surgeon to whom I was referred. Dr. Gates listened patiently as I relayed my predicament to him, hoping my face mask would hide my strained expression. "I know it will affect the prognosis and it'll be a much more involved surgery if I wait another five to six weeks. But I'm committed to Friends of the Smokies to raise this money, and I've already delayed the attempt because of the pandemic. I'm just going to deal with the risks and consequences, but I accept them," I explained.

It was instantly apparent that Dr. Gates would not berate me or try to guilt me into postponing my hike. Instead, he was fascinated with the prospect of merging an athletic endeavor with a cause he understood the importance of, especially since he enjoyed hiking, too.

He paused, excused himself from the room for a moment, and then returned. "What if I told you I could work you into my surgery schedule tomorrow afternoon? We still have a week before you start your hike. That gives us time to remove your cast the day before you hike and fit you with a custom molded splint. You won't need to start hand therapy until after your hike ends, and I think you'll be okay with the splint if you're very careful."

I accepted Dr. Gates' generous offer, amazed at my good fortune. When I returned the following day for surgery, the pre-operative nurse told me, "You must be pretty special for Dr. Gates to work you in like this."

"I'm not special, but the reason he worked me in is. I'm beyond appreciative of his kindness and compassion," I replied to her while blinking back tears of gratitude. Soon after, I drifted into the world of lost time under anesthesia. I woke up in recovery with a cast extending from my fingers to nearly the top of my forearm, eight days before we were to begin our hike.

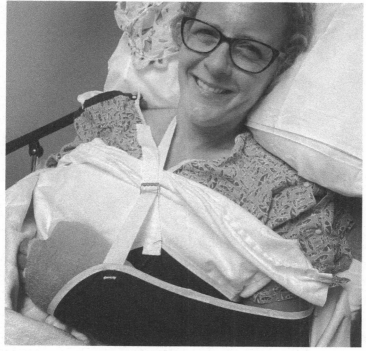

Eight days before the hike begins…

CHAPTER SIX

The Gauntlet

If you're gonna be dumb, you gotta be tough.

—ROGER ALAN WADE

Day 5—27.9 miles
(3098' gain, 7697' loss)

We started with a brisk walk on the nearly level Oconaluftee River Trail accompanied by the haunting cries of bugling bull elk nearby. We were mindful to not cross paths with one in the foggy darkness, fully aware of their power and speed.

It was one of three segments we'd hike throughout the course of the day—each longer than the previous one, all collectively adding up to one of our shortest mileage days. However, it was also one of our longest days logistically because of the driving times between trailheads, coupled with the fact that we were moving our "base camp" from Cherokee to Gatlinburg that evening.

This day also had a carrot dangling at the end. When we finished hiking, Larry, along with Paige and Wogene (two of my kids) were shuttling us from the Deep Creek trailhead back to our cars at the top of Thomas Divide Trail on Newfound Gap Road. I couldn't wait to see them in person. While we had FaceTimed daily, seeing them

32

would assuredly feed my soul in a more proper way. That and the calorie-laden Chick-fil-A meal they also promised to bring.

As we descended Thomas Divide Trail on our third and final segment of the day, I scolded myself for forgetting to add an extra water bottle to my backpack before we started an 11-mile dry stretch of trail. The day was warm and humid, and staying hydrated was paramount. When we were filtering water many hours later, I discovered that the extra bottle was there the whole time—I had placed it in a different location than I normally would.

Chris offered some of his water to me, but I declined. Unless I was desperate, I had an aversion to drinking after someone else, even Larry. Chris was the same way, and it was one of the many unusual characteristics of our personalities that aligned. Sometimes I felt Chris and I were long-lost twins rather than friends.

To keep my mind off thirst, we relived one of our favorite and most notorious hiking memories: The Gauntlet. It was a dress rehearsal of sorts that we executed six weeks prior to the start of our actual attempt on September 4. The Gauntlet consisted of hiking the first five days of our planned FKT routes to try them on for size and see how they felt.

Everything went well during The Gauntlet until our fifth and final day when we planned to hike four different segments, all separated by varying driving distances between trailheads. The last segment was a 12-mile stretch extending from Clingmans Dome northbound on the Appalachian Trail, ending at the Chimney Tops trailhead, after hiking Road Prong Trail, too.

In a last-minute decision, we hiked Road Prong and Chimney Tops Trails first, drove our waiting car from Chimney Tops up to Clingmans Dome, and then hiked south on the Appalachian Trail back to Road Prong's trailhead. Our reasoning was that we'd get the harder trails out of the way first, especially since we'd be hiking them in the dark.

Finally, after nearly twenty-four hours of hiking, which included the lengthy driving times we had underestimated, we finished the route at 4:30 a.m. At 3:00 a.m., when I discovered we had only hiked another half mile and I was certain we should have completed at least two, I said to Chris, exasperated, "I feel like we're on an episode of the Twilight Zone walking on some kind of hiking trail treadmill that won't ever let us get to the end!"

When we finally arrived at Chris' car and he opened his Crosstrek's rear hatch to place our backpacks in it, the noxious smell of the socks he had worn previously during the week—which had been festering in the heat of his car all day—hit us like a freight train. We both doubled over, hardly able to breathe from laughing so hard. Our efforts completely gutted us, and now we had to endure the foul odor while driving back to retrieve my car at Clingmans Dome.

If either of us had been alone, the scene may have triggered a less humorous reaction. But together as friends, it was hysterical. "At least the smell will keep us awake while you drive," I said to Chris when I finally composed myself, only to erupt in more peals of laughter as we drove back up the mountain.

Similar to the Tour de Le Conte, I viewed The Gauntlet as a proving ground for our compatibility during an extreme endeavor. That we were laughing uncontrollably after five days of hiking 186 miles—even after hiking for nearly twenty-four hours to finish the final day's route—was all the proof I needed to recognize the strength of our friendship and how it would weave into the story of our FKT.

Afterward, we changed our fifth day's route, and we shifted the last segment to the following day. It was not the first and it would not be the last time we needed to improvise, adapt and overcome throughout our journey. Our ability to do so would also prove to be a familiar theme to our success.

At day's end, Larry, Paige, and Wogene were walking towards us on Deep Creek Trail as we hiked our last mile. They were kind and didn't mention how bad I smelled after hiking all day in the heat when I pulled them to me in a group hug. It felt like five months, not five days, since I pulled out of our driveway, heading towards Cherokee.

It would be another week and a half before I saw them again in Gatlinburg, and I tried hard to keep my head and heart separated to stay focused on my goal. But just before we parted ways, I broke down unexpectedly. I wasn't sure if my tears stemmed from missing them or from gratitude. Probably a little of both. Either way, I was certain their love for me was the taproot beneath my strength and success so far.

As I drove away from them and crested the park's divide at Newfound Gap, crossing over into Tennessee, I exhaled deeply while looking at the landscape of North Carolina in my rearview mirror. I had accomplished the first five days without injury. I knew the race was far from won and that these first few days were just a warmup. But I also recognized the value of celebrating the minor victories and milestones along the way.

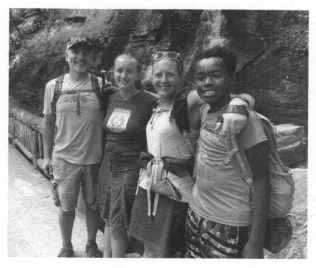

DAY 5: Larry, Paige, Nancy, and Wogene at Juney Whank Falls.

CHAPTER SEVEN

The Shoulders of Giants

One can never consent to creep when one feels an impulse to soar.

—HELEN KELLER

Day 6—33.2 miles
(5462' gain, 10,314' loss)

The previous evening, we settled into Buckberry Lodge, a solitary building sitting high above Gatlinburg. A victim of the extensive wildfires of 2016, Buckberry was once a premier destination in the area with multiple lodging options. Only this building escaped the fires that quickly burned 16,000 acres and consumed fourteen lives and more than 2,000 structures. It was the deadliest wildfire in the eastern United States since 1947.

We were grateful to the owners of the lodge for sponsoring our fundraiser by allowing us to stay for two weeks. Each of our units had a full kitchen, living room, and bathroom with a gloriously oversized bathtub in which I soaked my aching body most nights.

As comfortable as our accommodations were, I couldn't get comfortable when I crawled into bed. As soon as I would drift off to sleep, my sciatic nerve would jolt me awake, sending searing pain from my lower back, through my buttock, and into the back of my upper thigh. I hadn't experienced this kind of discomfort since the latter part of pregnancy with two of my children. Initially, I thought the hotel mattress in Cherokee caused it since it was firmer than mine at home, but now it was repeatable no matter where I slept.

I tried placing ice packs under my back and taking ibuprofen— otherwise known as "Vitamin I" in the hiking world. I also tried repositioning my body in various ways, including child's pose, my favorite Yoga stretch to ease tension in my normal, everyday life. But there was nothing normal about pushing one's body this hard each day, over and over. The only thing that eased the pain, ironically, was getting up and walking around the room.

After another night of far less sleep than I needed, Jamie drove us to Clingmans Dome at 5:00 a.m. where we would start another multi-segmented route with several drives between trailheads. As we were unloading our backpacks, we glimpsed a woman passing by in the dark. It only took a moment for both of us to connect the dots and recognize her face.

It was Sharon Spezia, a woman who had achieved legendary status in the Smokies community. Sharon had hiked the Smokies 900 Challenge nine times, starting when she was sixty years old. She even achieved the original FKT of the challenge in 2015, finishing all the trails in four months when she was sixty-five years old. She followed up this impressive feat by hiking another full map of the Smokies within the same calendar year. I had admired her from a distance for several years, and I couldn't believe my luck that I was about to introduce myself to her during our attempt.

"Are you Sharon?" I called out to her. She instantly gave us a glimpse of her good sense of humor. "No, I'm Sue," she replied, with a twinkle in her eye. She didn't let her fans down though, allowing us to take a photo with her.

She was heading out on an ambitious day hike with members of a local hiking group, and none of them had heard about our FKT attempt. When we told them we were going after the FKT, Sharon misunderstood and thought we were using a strange acronym to refer to hiking Forney Creek Trail, whose trailhead was close by. Or perhaps her sense of humor was just emerging again. It was hard to tell. But the one thing we knew was that Sharon impressed us.

After saying our goodbyes to Jamie, then to Sharon's hiking crew, we started our day with the route we shifted after the grueling Gauntlet. The feeling of being on a hiker treadmill never crossed my mind, and we made quick work of the miles.

We battled the tourist traffic that had accumulated since we started hiking that morning. I reminded myself that we were lucky to battle tourist traffic because it meant the park was open to visitors again. Four months prior, just weeks before we were scheduled to start our FKT attempt in the spring, the park closed in response to the COVID-19 pandemic. It was a setback and disappointment, especially not knowing when it would open. Just as worrisome, we also had to consider the possibility of it closing again once we started our FKT attempt. The park reopened by summer with no sign of shutting down again. Still, I held my breath. If 2020 taught me anything, it was to let go of expectations.

March 17, 2020

My car was packed and ready to go with several days' worth of food and camping gear. Chris and I were meeting for five days of high-mileage training hikes on the Tennessee side of the Smokies, priming our bodies with trial runs. The last time I had hiked this many days in a row was a year prior on our 7-day backpacking trip on the Benton MacKaye Trail, when we agreed to attempt the FKT together. I could only break free from my everyday obligations to hike once or twice weekly. This training period was critical.

Three days prior, Roy Cooper, North Carolina's governor, mandated all public schools to close their doors for in-person instruction and transition to a virtual learning platform. My kids were in shock. The abrupt departure from the daily interaction with their friends, coupled with the additional state mandates of reduced group sizes and quarantine measures, was akin to someone telling me I can't go hiking.

I'd soon realize this level of discomfort, too. Most of the public lands in our region, including Great Smoky Mountains National Park, eventually closed to visitors indefinitely to avoid overcrowding and increased transmission of the COVID-19 virus.

Paige was especially anxious. The night before I left to meet Chris, she broke down in tears and asked if I'd consider staying home. I hugged her and did my best to assuage her fears, telling her I'd cancel the hike while silently wrestling with my disappointment of bailing on our training hikes. Afterward, I went to my minivan and laid in the cot I had placed in the back of it. I wanted to test it out for comfort during our training since we had reservations in several frontcountry campgrounds throughout our attempt. I suspected the setup would provide more rest than a tent, and I was proud of the cozy nest I created for myself. But our plans would soon be thwarted when the park's campgrounds closed. Many remained that way for months, forcing us to rethink our lodging and look for hotels around the park instead.

I called Chris from the cot and told him the bad news. In typical fashion, he took it in stride. Chris and Jamie did not have children of their own, but they both had an exceptional awareness and understanding of parenting.

The next day, Chris headed out by himself for a training hike, but he turned back before he reached the trailhead. His text to me read, "The further I got away from home, the more I felt I was going the wrong way." We would meet for a day hike one week later, but it would be the last time we saw each other for nearly six weeks.

But now here we were, on our sixth day of the FKT attempt and the park's closure was all but a distant memory. We successfully navigated the inevitable traffic around Gatlinburg and hiked Twin Creeks Trail first, followed by Rainbow Falls and Bullhead trails which led us up and down Mount Le Conte once again. Our day ended on the Gatlinburg Trail, where Jamie was waiting to pick us up on the edge of the bustling town.

When we returned to Buckberry that evening, my left lower thigh was painful as I got out of my car. I limped to my room, suspicious that my muscles had tensed up during the drive—my body was quick

to let me know what it thought of my demands. A good night's rest—
hopefully more than the previous night—would be just the thing to
recalibrate everything.

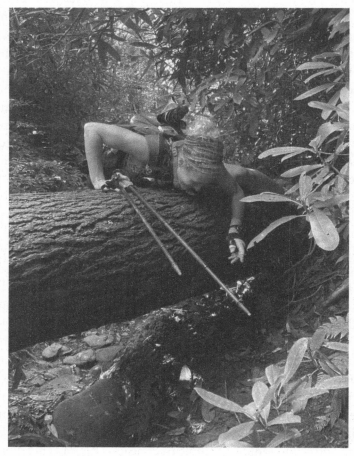

DAY 6: On Road Prong Trail.

CHAPTER EIGHT

Thunder Thighs

The words you speak become the house you live in.

—RUMI

Day 7—34.2 miles
(5455' gain, 6435' loss)

The previous night, my thigh pain didn't persist once I was off my feet, but sciatica continued to plague me. I woke up and only felt a slight twinge of discomfort in my thigh as I descended the stairs from my second-level room at Buckberry Lodge. "Thank God that's better," I thought to myself. The last thing I needed was an escalating injury to slow us down on a 34-mile day.

We had hiked this day's route over the summer, and we knew it to be a relatively easy one, despite the long mileage to get us from start to finish. Who it wasn't easy on, however, was Jamie. She would end up shuttling us three different times throughout the day, and she even took on the stinky task of washing our filthy hiking clothes in Townsend at a laundromat between her drives to meet us. I suspected Jamie would not think Chris' socks were as funny as we did the night we finished The Gauntlet.

As predicted by our previous training hike, the miles went down smooth—until they didn't anymore—at least for me. My thigh became increasingly tight and painful throughout the day, but especially during our final eight miles down Cove Mountain Trail.

Five o'clock finally arrived, which I had previously designated as "Hiker Happy Hour." Every day around the same time, I'd pull out my most coveted snack—Cheetos—to munch on while we hiked. Even the temporary endorphin rush that my salty, artificial orange, finger-lickin' good snack provided wasn't taking my mind off my discomfort.

"Something's not quite right with my left leg. I'm not sure what's causing it," I finally admitted to Chris.

"Do you want to stop and stretch?" he asked.

"Yeah, I guess I should to see if it helps. I felt a twinge of similar pain last night, but it's worse now."

We stopped and I stretched, not knowing even which stretches might help. Deep squats were my favorite thing to do after a long hike, since they loosened up the tension in my thighs. Except now I was having immense difficulty squatting. Even when I stopped to pee, I had to improvise my normal stance of sinking low to the ground to make myself as inconspicuous as possible. My tensed leg was now forcing me to stand in a half upright, half squatting position as I emptied my bladder.

I hoped that getting off my feet overnight would resolve the issue again, as it had the previous night. By the end of the hike, however, I was side stepping down Cove Mountain Trail. I could hardly bend my left knee going downhill without it seizing in pain. Our pace slowed to a crawl, but Chris was patient and kind. If he was concerned about where this injury was headed, he didn't show it.

I remembered something Chris had told me on a training hike that summer—words I didn't want to remember for fear they were coming true as I hobbled down Cove Mountain. "If either of us gets an overuse injury during the FKT, it will probably happen in the first two weeks. If we can get through that time frame successfully, I'll feel really good about both of us finishing this."

My thighs were a blessing and a curse. As a child, my younger brother once called me "Thunder Thighs" because of their size (to be fair, he was insecure about his much leaner build and I took advantage by dubbing him "Chicken Legs").

"You're just big boned and strong as an ox. Nothing wrong with that," my dad would tell me afterward. I later learned about different body types in school and pegged myself as mostly mesomorphic, meaning I had a muscular, stocky build--'mostly,' because my eating habits softened the look.

My mostly mesomorphic frame powered me up mountains, but I didn't always return the favor of its strength with my food choices. My sweet tooth was strong, and sugar was my medicine in times of stress—which was almost every day while raising three children. I pondered if this shortcoming of willpower was factoring into my injury, since I often carried a little more weight than I should. "If it will just go away, I won't ever touch another M&M," I lied to myself.

When Jamie pulled up at Sugarlands Visitor Center to take us back to Buckberry Lodge for the evening, she noticed the quiet tension in the car as we drove out of the park. "Y'all aren't your usual chatty selves. What's going on?"

"It's me," I replied. "I'm dealing with some kind of pain in my thigh, but I think getting a good night's sleep is gonna make it all better." But I wasn't as confident as I had been the previous night.

That evening, I took a bath, willing the hot water to scour away my pain. Dr. Google helped me research my symptoms and what might be wrong. It was far from an ideal way to problem solve, but it was the only medical advice I had time for, no matter how inaccurate it might be. A pulled or torn quadriceps muscle seemed to be the most likely culprit. I had been battling knee pain for the past week too, so referred pain from my knee could also be the cause. Whatever it was, it needed to get better overnight. We couldn't afford for me to continue with Chris on this journey if I could only cover one mile per hour.

CHAPTER NINE

Trouble in Paradise

If you are going through hell, keep going.
—WINSTON CHURCHILL

Day 8—30.6 miles
(6614' gain, 6618' loss)

I woke up the next morning, and once again, the overnight rest had eased most of the pain in my leg. We hiked Grapeyard Ridge Trail first, still in the dark, laughing about the likelihood of coming across a tiger that had gone missing from the Knoxville Zoo. It was good to be back in our routine with focus and intent, but never too serious to laugh, especially if we could add our own imaginative spin to a story.

As we headed up Trillium Gap Trail a few hours later, the pain in my leg returned with a vengeance. Stretching helped, but the relief was brief and minimal. I had a pocket of cell reception, so I texted a friend and physical therapist, Eric Yarrington, hoping he'd help me troubleshoot the problem.

As expected, it was difficult for him to assist me through a text conversation. I gathered the courage and asked if he would meet me in his office that evening to examine me. "I'm more than willing to pay you an after hours fee," I wrote to him. Knowing Eric, he'd never accept it, though. Without hesitation, he agreed to give up his Friday evening to examine my leg. Once again, I was touched by the kindness and compassion of members of my region's medical community.

But Chris and I still had many miles and hours to hike before I could make the hour and a half drive to Eric's office in Waynesville. I promised him I would be there by 8:00 p.m., at the latest. I wasn't sure how I was going to get through our route and stick to that timeline, but I'd figure out a way—even if it meant turning up the dial on my pain level to walk faster.

To add insult to injury, my GI system was responding negatively to stress, and I was experiencing sharp cramps. I had been battling abdominal problems from the extreme demands I was putting on my body, but this took it to the next level of discomfort, and my stomach churned in urgent protest.

"Using the bathroom" when hikers need to void their bowels rather than their bladder doesn't involve any kind of "room" at all in the backcountry. By adhering to Leave No Trace principles, pooping was a more involved process than tucking away behind a bush to squat or stand and pee on the ground's surface. I searched hastily for a secluded place off the trail to dig a proper 6-inch cat hole in one of the most popular areas of the Smokies. I desperately hoped it would only amount to a onetime pit stop and that my leg would allow me to squat low enough to hide myself from hikers on the nearby trails.

After my detour, we ascended Trillium Gap Trail to Mount Le Conte's summit, only to turn around and descend it again, but not without another urgent side trip to the restrooms the lodge kept open for hikers. As we descended the mountain, a torrential downpour caught us off guard, flooding the trail and making it look like a small stream rather than a footpath. The challenge of hiking in the rain at least took my mind off the pain. I needed to focus on every step so as not to slip and do more damage to my already compromised leg.

"These are the times you're going to have to dig deep to earn this FKT," I reminded myself. I reflected on what I learned during my natural childbirth class when I was pregnant—that pain is often a necessary precursor to great reward. I knew the FKT endeavor would not end without experiencing higher levels of physical pain than I'd likely ever known, short of enduring labor without medication. But the pain of childbirth only lasted a day or so. If my leg pain didn't let up, it would last for weeks before we finished.

"You reveled in childbirth, Nancy, pain and all. Just pretend you're giving birth over and over, every single day until the end," I mused. The thought of delivering a baby every day for the next three weeks and having twenty-one children to raise afterward was welcome comic relief as I fumbled through the pouring rain. Undoubtedly, this effort was easier compared to that!

By the time we reached Brushy Mountain Trail, I could no longer distract myself from my discomfort. My leg was on fire and my pain was the worst it had been since the problem started two days prior. We still had six miles to reach our cars, and the trail had transitioned from looking like a small creek to a pigpen. Recent horse activity on Brushy Mountain had annihilated the trail tread, leaving a muddy mess in its wake.

If I wasn't sliding down a slick stretch of mud, fighting to stay upright, I was pulling my foot out of a deep pit of it. The suction effect created by the thick mud pulled my foot out of my shoe several times. I was also side stepping again to avoid the pain. It was an infuriatingly slow endeavor. The silver lining to the continued downpour was that Chris couldn't hear the near constant outburst of expletives pouring from my mouth.

After an eternity, the rain tapered off as we were nearing the bottom of the mountain. We could talk and hear each other again, so it was time to war game the next two days' worth of routes, which included our only overnight stay in the backcountry.

The following morning, Aidan, my 17-year-old son, Isaac, my 16-year-old nephew, and Dawson Wheeler, a new friend and supporter of our attempt, were scheduled to meet up and take the boat shuttle across Fontana Lake. They would hike in and meet us at campsite 82 beside Hazel Creek, where we'd all camp for the night.

Chris and I would then wake up early and hike our next route, while our support team would take the boat shuttle back across the lake. The help from our team would eliminate the need for us to carry extra backpacking gear on two of our most aggressive routes.

It was easy to shuffle the deck with many of our routes, but this one involved the help of two teens who were expected to be back in school, albeit virtually, on Monday morning. Dawson was coming from Chattanooga, so we didn't want to lose his help either. We agreed to wait and hear what Eric said before making the final decision. But I was already hellbent on sticking to the original plan, assuming I wouldn't hold Chris back.

"I'm planning to come back to Gatlinburg tonight after Eric works some magic on my leg, so we should plan to start on time tomorrow morning. Would you mind getting in touch with Dawson and letting him know what's going on?" I asked Chris in a voice as determined as I could make it. I knew my feigned confidence didn't fool him, but we both recognized the value of an optimistic outlook.

"Yep, I'm happy to do it. Let's just figure out the best thing to do once you see Eric. If we have to change things up and do an easier route tomorrow instead, it'll be ok and we'll make it all work." Chris replied. Once again, he took a stressful situation in stride—his calm and supportive demeanor held my fragile state of mind up to a light I couldn't clearly see on my own.

I drove to Waynesville in another downpour—the mood of the mountains reflecting mine. I knew I needed to prepare myself for bad news from Eric. What if I had torn a ligament or had done something that would continue to get worse? I couldn't fathom only making it eight days into the attempt before having to pull the plug on my efforts. Chris and I had spoken at length during our training about the potential for one of us becoming injured. We agreed that the other person should continue on, attempting to earn the FKT by themselves. But more than anything, we wanted to be by each other's side at the end.

Eric examined me and determined that I had injured one of my quadriceps muscles—my *vastus medialis*—just as I had suspected. "You can keep hiking on it and modify your gait like you've been doing until you potentially can't hike anymore from the pain. But there's no reason you can't keep trying if you choose to," he told me. His words were all I needed to give the next day's intended plan the green light.

He performed dry needling in the injured area of my leg. As the needles entered the belly of my muscle and it spasmed in response, I cherished the pain. I knew it meant I stood a chance of getting better. Eric also taught me a taping technique to provide more stability and hopefully lessen my pain while the muscle healed. When I stepped down off the exam table, I felt somewhat more at ease about my predicament—and I swear my leg felt a little better, too.

My family was waiting for me at home, where I stopped on the way out to see them for a few minutes and to pick up the Chick-fil-A salad and milkshake that I had requested for dinner. The roles of mother and child were temporarily reversed with my two younger children. I felt like the child being nurtured and cared for instead of the other way around.

Wogene gave me an enormous hug—a physical gesture usually far removed from his teenage comfort zone. Paige took the salad container out of my hand and cut its contents into more manageable pieces to eat, recognizing that I'd struggle with the task while wearing my hand splint.

Aidan had his backpack loaded up, ready to go early the next morning. I was nervous about him finding his way to the marina to catch the boat shuttle, but I knew he was determined to do all he could to help me succeed. A text he sent to me the day prior further validated it: "Hey mom I love you. Wanted to let you know that I'm so proud to call you my mom. I saw your insta post. 242 MILES IN 7 DAYS!!!! Strongest woman I will ever know."

Larry didn't question my choice to return to Gatlinburg and proceed with the next day's route as planned. Some spouses might have protested their significant other driving nearly two hours late at night in poor weather, especially given the day's events. But over the course of our 20-year marriage, Larry had developed a sixth sense for which battles to choose with me. Plus, I knew his confidence in my abilities outweighed any concerns he might have—and it made me love him even more.

I promised my family, "If this injury gets worse and takes me off the trail, you have my word that I'll be mature about it and not burden you with my disappointment. You've all sacrificed so much to allow me this opportunity, and I owe you that."

It was an unintentional empty promise, and words that I knew I would regret speaking to them should my failure come to fruition. I would need my family's support and compassion to help guide me through the loss of a goal I had worked so hard and for so long to achieve.

But with all my heart, I also believed that I wouldn't need to make good on that promise. What I had lacked throughout my life in natural athletic abilities, I had made up for in determination and perseverance. There were certain injuries that could force me off the trail, but a badly strained muscle would not be one of them.

Still, as I was walking out to the driveway to get in my minivan, I felt acutely absurd. Parents in our quiet mountain town were likely loading up their own minivans that evening with folding camp chairs and special snacks for Saturday morning soccer games, not limping to them in a quest to set a nearly 1,000-mile speed record in the back-country with an injury. In that moment, I wasn't sure if I was setting a good or a bad example for my kids with my audacious act anymore. I was too far in though, and there was no turning back.

So I waved goodbye to them standing in the opening of our garage, rolling down the window to tell them I loved them one more time. And I knew they loved me as much in return—more than enough to excuse my behavior if it disappointed them. I arrived at Buckberry Lodge a few minutes shy of midnight. Exhausted, I climbed into bed with all my hiking clothes still on and woke up three hours later to start the next day.

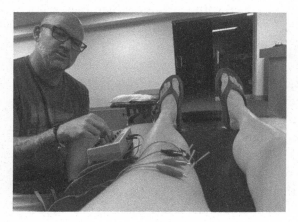

DAY 8, evening: Eric Yarrington, PT, dry needling Nancy's leg.

CHAPTER TEN

Hell on Hazel Creek

Here is the world. Beautiful and terrible things will happen.
Don't be afraid.

—FREDERICK BUECHNER

Day 9—33.4 miles
(7694' gain, 6777' loss)

My phone's alarm jolted me awake, and for a moment, I couldn't remember how I ended up in the bed. I limped to the bathroom to get ready for the day, ignoring the voice in my head telling me I was crazy to think I could keep up with Chris. Less than twelve hours prior, I wasn't even able to take a step without wincing in nearly debilitating pain and slowing our pace significantly.

I had done all I could do to speed up my recovery, short of taking time off to let my leg rest. I knew I had to at least attempt the day's hike, especially since our support team was heading out to start their trek into campsite 82 with our overnight gear. We'd rendezvous at the campsite in the evening, convening from opposite directions.

As we started our route up West Prong Trail, my leg still hurt. But unlike the day before, it wasn't hindering my ability to move efficiently. I suspected that would change as the day wore on, as it had the last two days. But I'd take as much of a reprieve as I could get.

Within the first ten miles of our hike, we encountered dozens of hikers along Bote Mountain Trail and the Appalachian Trail. They were heading to Rocky Top, a familiar mountaintop in the Smokies, to celebrate the start of the University of Tennessee football season. Many of them had been following our efforts through social media, and it was exciting to put names with faces that I had only known virtually until then. Their enthusiasm and positive energy were contagious—the encounters took my mind off my leg and bolstered my confidence.

Later, as we were walking along a high ridgeline on the Appalachian Trail, I took my phone out of airplane mode to make sure Aidan hadn't texted me with some sort of snafu catching the boat shuttle to Hazel Creek. No word from Aidan. Instead, I received a message from Rick Morrow, one of our hiking friends, informing us that campsite 82 was closed. Chris checked his email since the reservation was under his name, but the park service hadn't sent him a closure notification—a standard operating procedure.

Our small pocket of cell reception disappeared quickly as we continued walking. The only reasonable course was to forge ahead, meet with our crew as scheduled, and see if the campsite had a closure notification posted in it. If it did, we'd just move further down the trail a few more miles to campsite 83. Not ideal, as it would make a long day even longer, but at least we'd have a head start on our mileage the following day.

A few miles later, we arrived at the junction of the Appalachian Trail and Welch Ridge. There was a park-issued sign stapled to the trailhead that read, "Hazel Creek Trail closed from Welch Ridge Trail to the junction with Cold Spring Gap Trail until further notice. Do not put yourself or others at risk by ignoring this closure."

It was a common occurrence for backcountry campsites to close temporarily in the park. This was usually in response to increased bear activity, stemming from careless campers leaving food scraps in fire pits or around the campsite; however, the closure of a trail was not common. Adding even more complexity to the situation, campsite 82 was on the closed stretch of trail.

We had scant cell reception on the ridge again. Chris called Jamie to see if the park had notified her about the campsite closure, since she was an emergency contact for us on the permit. I could hear Jamie's voice through the speaker on Chris' phone. "Yes, it's all over social media and the news today," she explained. "A man's body was being eaten by a bear in campsite 82. That's why the trail is closed."

My mind immediately jumped to a worst-case scenario—a member of our support team could be the "man" Jamie was referring to. I had to lean against a tree to stay upright. Adrenaline surged through my body, and I felt as if the weight of the world was resting squarely on my shoulders, pressing me down into the earth. The imagery my brain conjured up was terrifying.

"Oh my God, what if it was one of our people?!" I said, panic-stricken. "What the hell is going on? This can't be happening!"

I had always harbored the fear that one of my seemingly benign choices would put my children on a trajectory of injury or death—worried that if I drove a certain route over another, it might put us in the path of a drunk driver; or, as a sleep-deprived mother, I feared leaving one of them in their car seat during a sweltering summer day. Yet, never in a million years would I have imagined innocently putting my son in harm's way with an aggressive black bear in the Smokies. But here I was, believing my worst nightmare might have come true.

"Jamie, are you sure?! I have a panicked mother standing beside me who is very worried about her son right now." She quickly answered, "No, Aidan is fine! They're all fine! This happened last night. The bear is dead—the rangers shot it today when they found it still feeding on the man's body. Some hikers walked up on the scene yesterday and alerted the park last night when they found an area with cell reception."

Chris hung up with Jamie, and we stood together in shock, still processing her words. Things like this were almost unheard of in the Smokies. The only fatality from a bear attack since the park's inception was in 2000, twenty years prior. Two bears killed a 50-year-old woman, Glenda Bradley, on Little River Trail.

Lane was hiking elsewhere, so we couldn't reach him to troubleshoot the situation. I called Larry and discovered he had been communicating with Aidan through our Garmin InReach, a GPS device that allowed 2-way messaging through satellites. Larry could tell that their communication had gaps though, and we later discovered that Aidan was walking around with the unit dangling from a lanyard around his neck, making it more difficult for messages to transmit.

Larry and I shared extensive details with Aidan about the plan to provide support for us. But we had inadvertently neglected to teach him how to send messages through the InReach, including the importance of keeping the unit stationary during the process. All he knew was how to press the SOS button if he had a genuine emergency and needed help. Despite the gaps in communication, Larry knew the most important facts: that our crew was safe and had been redirected to campsite 83 by park rangers who were in the Hazel Creek area.

Thick clouds were closing in and it started raining, so I hung up with Larry. Our cell reception was deteriorating with the increased fog, but eventually we got a call out to the backcountry office. We received a recording that they were closed for the day. It dawned on me that we could call 911 and be transferred to the park's dispatch center. They transferred us to a backcountry ranger, and we explained our predicament.

The ranger knew who we were since our FKT attempt was receiving a good bit of publicity. We pled her mercy by explaining that our support team, including my son, was waiting for us at campsite 83 and that we had no overnight gear with us. We needed to get down there, and our intended route along the closed trail was the quickest way to do it. The ranger sternly informed us we could not hike the closed portion of Hazel Creek Trail and that we could reach campsite 83 via Welch Ridge and Cold Springs Gap trails, a path that would add seven extra miles to our day.

She also encouraged us to consider hiking out to Clingmans Dome and have someone meet us, to take us somewhere safe for the night and figure out our next steps. Even though the rangers were fairly confident that they had euthanized the correct bear, they couldn't be sure without further testing, she told us.

Her words implied it wasn't clear if the man had been the victim of a bear attack or if he had died of another cause and was being scavenged upon by the bear. She also relayed that more bears may have been involved and might return to the area to look for the man's body. "I personally wouldn't want to be anywhere along Hazel Creek tonight," she said.

"What do you want to do?!" Chris asked me with exasperation in his voice and tears in his eyes. I had never seen Chris like this. His cool headed, calm outlook was one of his greatest strengths. It was oddly comforting to witness his concern and emotion about our situation. While he was surely concerned about reaching Aidan, Isaac and Dawson too, he recognized and was reacting in response to my deeper connection to it. All he had to do was replace Aidan's face with Jamie's to relate to what I was feeling.

"We have to keep hiking," I said through tears. "I have to get to Aidan. I need to know he's really okay, and I know he'll worry about me if I don't show up." So, we hiked on, into the rain and fog towards campsite 83, tethered tightly by the bonds of empathy and friendship while darkness quickly descended.

There was an eerie vibe to the woods as we walked along Welch Ridge. We were close to the area where a man had tragically died the night before, possibly from a bear attack. There is power in numbers with uninvited wild animal encounters though, and I suspected Chris was as grateful for my physical presence as I was for his.

I was also grateful for him when a tiny insect abruptly flew deep into my ear canal. "Chris, I need to stop," I said urgently. "A bug just flew into my ear canal and I think it's stuck in there!"

I couldn't believe it. We were already hiking seven additional miles at night, in a potentially dangerous area. Now I was about to be driven insane by the loud buzzing of an insect in my ear. It felt like we were in another episode of the Twilight Zone—or maybe it was a horror movie this time.

I stuck my pinky finger into my ear as far as I could, attempting to squash the bug against my ear canal before it went any deeper. But I couldn't reach it. "Aaaah—it keeps buzzing! This is awful!" I shrieked. "Hold still," Chris said calmly. "Do you care if I blow in your ear really hard? Maybe I can force it out like an air compressor."

"I don't care what you do, I just want it out!" I exclaimed, trying my best to hold still when it started buzzing again.

What a sight we must have been if a bear was lurking somewhere watching us—Chris' face, an inch from my ear, blowing short puffs of air as forcefully as he could, while I was blankly staring off into space, doing my best not to panic when the bug started buzzing again.

Blowing in my ear while stretching my ear canal to its limit didn't work; nor did shining a flashlight in it, hoping the light might attract the bug to fly towards it and out of my ear. Chris' quick mind was already a step ahead, though. He pulled a Q-tip out of his backpack. "Here, see if you can dig it out with this." I inserted the Q-tip in my ear to the point of discomfort, but the only thing I withdrew was a big blob of ear wax. "Ew, this is so gross—I hardly ever clean my ears out! And why do you have Q-tips in your backpack, anyway?" I said, half laughing, the levity lessening my panic.

"It's okay. I'm not bothered by seeing your ear wax. And I always carry Q-tips in my backpack," Chris said, laughing a little too. At least my disregard for hygiene was providing some humor to our situation. There was still the insect to contend with, though, and my nerves were feeling more frayed by the second.

"Wait a minute, I don't hear it anymore," I said. I started wondering if I had hallucinated the entire ordeal in my sleep-deprived state from the night before. Chris shined the light into my ear to see if he could visualize anything. "I see it! At least part of its legs and body. I think you must have crushed it with the Q-tip," he said excitedly. He pulled the remnants out with another Q-tip. "Oh my God, what else can go wrong today?" I asked incredulously. "I shouldn't be tempting fate by asking that—never mind," I quickly answered.

By the time we reached the short out-and-back trail to High Rocks, a rocky outcropping where a fire tower once stood, my leg was in pain again. I was moving more slowly, and to make matters worse, the weather continued to worsen. It was now rainy, foggy, *and* windy— the perfect trifecta for a potential fall and injury. Chris could hardly see the trail in front of him, both from the fog and the overgrowth of late summer. The silver lining was that it forced him to move more slowly.

When we arrived at High Rocks, we were not in the right frame of mind to take requisite fun photos of each other sitting on the metal stool—all that remained of the fire tower besides the dilapidated caretaker's cabin behind us in the woods. Plus, it was completely dark. The revelation of having cell reception in this exposed location was far more appealing, so we called our spouses. I was eager to hear if Larry could successfully send a message to Aidan, letting him know we would arrive much later than expected but that we were safe.

When Larry told me he sent a message but he didn't receive one back from Aidan, I broke down in tears of frustration. The ranger's foreboding words echoed in my head—"I wouldn't want to be anywhere along Hazel Creek tonight." I just wanted to know our crew was okay, but we still had to descend Cold Springs Gap Trail to reach them, one of the most rocky and demanding trails in the entire park.

Mercifully, as we descended Cold Springs Gap, the weather improved. By the time we reached the notoriously tough stretch of trail that's covered in permanently wet and rocky boulders, we could actually move faster than we had in the rain and fog. I was grateful and kept reminding myself that we were on the home stretch.

As we descended towards Hazel Creek and I could hear it flowing in the distance, my nerves returned. The ranger we had spoken to previously had told us, "The water crossing on Hazel Creek might be high from the rain we've had over the last twenty-four hours. It's wide and can get dangerous, so stick together and be careful."

I knew the list of exceptionally dangerous unbridged water crossings in the Smokies by heart, and this one was on it. I had a healthy respect—and fear—of the power of swift water currents. I just hoped my injured leg didn't limit my ability to cross it safely.

We saw lights in the distance as we drew closer to the creek. We wondered if the park might position rangers overnight in the area, in case a bear emerged showing aggressive tendencies.

When we reached the creek's bank, I could tell the people on the other side weren't rangers. The bright headlamps shining at us hid their faces, but they were wearing hiking attire, not NPS uniforms. I wondered if it was our support crew, waiting for us to ensure we forded the creek safely, but the creek was too wide and loud to see or hear the people well.

Crossing the swollen creek was easier than I expected. When we stepped onto the bank on the opposite side, three strangers greeted us. They were camping at campsite 83 and had met our crew. They sensed Aidan's concern about our whereabouts when we didn't show up on time, especially when he told them I was battling a leg injury, so they came looking for us.

Shortly after they left camp, Larry's message came through to Aidan on the InReach. Aidan and Isaac ran after the men as they were heading down the trail, "My dad messaged me and said my mom and Chris are coming down Cold Springs Gap Trail now." So the trio headed to the creek and waited for us there.

Their kindness humbled me as we walked the final two miles to the campsite together in the dark. We weren't sure how strong of hikers they were, but they were going to have to be fast if they wanted to keep up with me. Even my injured leg didn't have the power to slow me down anymore. I was on a singularly focused mission—to hug my son and hold him tight. They kept our pace, and we arrived in camp just after 11:00 p.m.

I instantly recognized a red puffy jacket in the near distance. "Aidan!" I called out while jogging up to embrace him. My firstborn son was practically an adult now and towered over me in height, but all I could see was my sweet, tow-headed little boy grinning back at me. My world was back on its axis.

I hugged Isaac too, and then mistakenly said hello to another camper who I thought was Dawson. "I'm over here," Dawson said. I laughed when I realized my mistake. "Oh, there you are—sorry about that! It's so nice to finally meet you, and I can't apologize enough for the mess we've put you in."

Dawson and I had never met in person. Well known in the outdoor community and the founder of a popular outdoor retailer in Chattanooga, he had decades of achievements and accolades attached to his name. His most endearing quality, however, was his heart of gold.

Through the power of social media and connections in the Smokies community, we had gotten to know each other virtually through Kristi Parsons, a well-loved photographer in the Smokies, whose acquaintance I had made long before. Kristi assured me that Dawson would be the perfect person to ask to accompany Aidan and Isaac, and I knew I could trust her opinion.

We made our way into camp to make a quick dinner—realizing neither of us had eaten anything substantial in hours. Our crew surrounded us while we ate. They relayed how their day unfolded once they stepped off the boat that had carried them across Fontana Lake.

As they were hiking along Hazel Creek Trail that morning, utility terrain vehicles (UTV) carrying several park rangers drove up behind them, traveling in the same direction. The rangers stopped and inquired about their destination. Dawson pulled out his backcountry permit which verified their park-approved destination for the evening—campsite 82. The rangers exchanged troubled glances before telling them they would need to stay in campsite 83 instead, which they would pass about three miles prior to 82.

Dawson asked why, and the female ranger replied, "We're doing some trail maintenance." Dawson didn't buy it, especially when he noticed their rifles. "Trail maintenance? I don't see any shovels or tools though." There was a pause before the ranger answered. "It's an evolving situation, sir. Unfortunately, we can't tell you anything more at this point."

Dawson astutely read between the lines and knew there was more than trail maintenance happening along Hazel Creek that day. He was suspicious that the park service might be responding to a tip about ginseng hunters. Such poachers were an ongoing problem in the park, illegally digging the plant's roots to sell on the black market.

Eventually, our crew saw a UTV pass them again in the opposite direction, carrying something very large under a tarp with bloodstains on the side of the vehicle. The rangers hung signs in the area as well, announcing the closure of Hazel Creek Trail because of aggressive bear activity.

The rangers never disclosed what happened at campsite 82 to anyone camping along Hazel Creek. They warned the campers that the entire trail would likely close later in the day, but they eventually retracted the statement and told them they could stay in campsite 83 for the evening.

While Aidan and Isaac were out of earshot, we filled Dawson in about the man being scavenged. There was no reason for the boys to hear, and I knew it would rattle Aidan. A couple of years prior on a school trip, he had camped at a different backcountry site in the park. That night, he woke up to the sound of two bears in the campsite. His teacher was a certified instructor for Leave No Trace (LNT) and had educated the students on LNT principles for the trip. They did an excellent job of abiding by them, even cleaning up litter left behind by prior campers.

Litter is a magnet for ursine visitors in campsites though, and the two bears had likely discovered it prior to that evening. Aidan didn't sleep a wink under his tarp. He worried the bears might become frustrated with the lack of trash and decide to snack on a 13-year-old boy instead. The experience unnerved him for future backpacking trips.

After we ate our dinner, I limped into the darkness to change into my sleeping clothes. I used a large cage on the edge of the campsite to steady myself while I pulled on my leggings. The cage was a trap used to control the population of non-native, invasive wild hogs in the park. But this one had long been neglected. I exhaled a deep sigh and looked upwards towards the heavens. "Mama, what a day. Thank you for watching over Aidan, Isaac and Dawson...and Chris and me, too," I whispered.

Aidan had pitched my tent before we arrived, but I slept in the 4-person tent he and Isaac were sharing. If an aggressive bear was still in the area and came to visit our campsite, I wanted to be close to them. I knew I was defenseless, but I never underestimated the inherent 'mother bear' instinct that lived inside me—the one I knew

I could call on at a moment's notice, even while exhausted, to protect my own—just like my mom was still doing for me.

Eventually, my body's fatigue outpaced my racing mind, and I slipped in and out of a restless sleep.

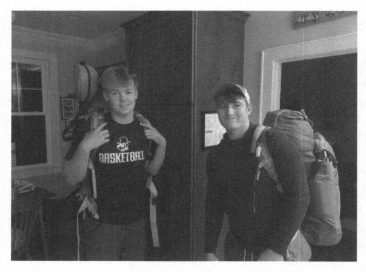

DAY 9: Isaac (left) and Aidan heading out to Hazel Creek in the morning.

CHAPTER ELEVEN

Forney Creek!

A man who has been through bitter experiences and travelled far
enjoys even his sufferings after a time.

—HOMER, *THE ODYSSEY*

Day 10—29.9 miles
(7553' gain, 3581' loss)

Aidan, Isaac, and Dawson were sleeping soundly when we started hiking. It was dark still, but the sun would peek over the mountains soon enough, facilitating their safe passage out of the woods and back to the boat shuttle across Fontana Lake. Our route would take us in the opposite direction on the same trail we dreaded hiking down the night before—Cold Springs Gap. Eventually we'd make a long ascent up Forney Creek Trail with its many wide, swift, and potentially deep creek crossings, to end at Clingmans Dome.

As we were climbing up Cold Springs Gap, we saw some hikers ahead of us, which wasn't a typical sight on this remote trail. As we got closer, we recognized one of them as an acquaintance of Jamie and Chris'—another US Air Force veteran, Dave Wallace. He was hiking with a friend, and this was the second time we had run into them in the Smokies over the last few months.

The Smokies community felt very small sometimes, despite the vastness of the park's acreage. They had spent the night in campsite

61

83 too, after being rerouted from campsite 82. The world felt even smaller, realizing we had all chosen the same campsite on the same night that one of the strangest incidents in park history occurred.

We continued up the mountain, then turned around and descended via Bear Creek Trail, and then finally started our 12-mile ascent of Forney Creek Trail. The creek crossings were deeper than normal from recent rains, but still manageable. We were both in good spirits, and the trail was kind to us with its gentle ascent until the last four miles, when it pitched more steeply.

Chris hollered out, "Forney Creeeek!" multiple times throughout the climb. The words spilling from his mouth were strong and confident, initially. But by day's end, he was dragging his poles behind him while staggering up the trail in an exaggerated fashion, whimpering the words. It made me laugh harder each time he did it—the 'slap happy' phase of our day had officially kicked in.

My leg injury didn't bother me as much when we ascended. While planning our routes, we asked Lane to set them up to descend as much as possible, thinking it would minimize how much we taxed our muscles. It was skewed logic though, as hiking downhill required strength too. It was also more jarring on our joints to hike downhill. I suspected our well-intentioned plan had contributed to my injury, so I was happy for a day that required us to ascend over twice as much as we descended.

We grew quieter in the last couple of miles, both ready for our feet to touch the pavement of Clingmans Dome parking area, where Jamie would meet us to take us back down to Gatlinburg. Despite the energy we had already exerted, when we started up Forney Ridge Trail our strides still outpaced every other hiker on the popular path. We had just hiked nearly thirty miles from one of the lowest points in the park to the very highest, and I could still hike at an efficient pace—proof that I was getting stronger, despite my injury.

We approached the junction of Forney Ridge Trail and the spur trail that branched off to the right from it. The spur trail would lead us to the parking area in another quarter mile. My mind's eye saw Susan Clements ahead of us, continuing on past the spur trail. Her gaze was probably focused on her feet to avoid tripping on the big rocks that covered the trail. It was a mistake plenty of tired hikers made in this exact spot, ending up on the Appalachian Trail a half mile later. Susan just didn't figure out she needed to backtrack quickly enough.

Minutes after hearing search teams had found her mother's body, her daughter, Elizabeth, ran to this point on the trail. She told her fiancé, David, who was following her, "I need to go down in the woods. I need to walk down this trail. I need to see where she made the wrong turn." David chased her, pleading with her not to continue. But Elizabeth, inconsolable and consumed by the shock of just learning her mother was dead, continued her sprint into the woods. "I knew her body was down there somewhere, and I was just screaming, Mom! Mom! Mom!" Elizabeth explained mournfully, her pain leaping through my computer screen and into me. I would carry it with me long after I finished watching her videos. No matter how tired I was during our FKT, I never lost sight of what Susan went through that night and how much pain her family would endure long afterwards.

As we climbed the last steps to the parking lot, we saw Jamie standing above us at the top, taking our picture. She earned her "Trail Angel of the Year" badge when we discovered not one, two, or three, but four different cold drinks waiting for each of us in the car, packed in a cooler: chocolate milk, grape soda, orange soda, and lemonade. Choosing one of them was the toughest decision I made the entire day. I decided I had enough challenges over the last forty-eight hours to justify two—possibly even three—of them. Chocolate milk, orange soda, and lemonade never tasted so good.

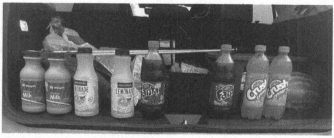

DAY 10: The bounty of drinks.

CHAPTER TWELVE

The Itsy Bitsy Spider

Hang on to your hat. Hang on to your hope.
And wind the clock, for tomorrow is another day."

—E.B. WHITE

Day 11—30.7 miles
(5883' gain, 6421' loss)

"I hate Old Settlers Trail," I whined. "It's soooo boring!" My sleep deprived state was making me irrational and grouchy. Collectively, I had only gotten about twelve hours of shuteye over the last three nights. Chris and I could both function well, at least physically, on little sleep. A chronic insomniac, I spent many nights wishing I had a toggle switch in my brain that I could turn to the "off" position. The only perk to the affliction was that it conditioned me for reduced sleep during the FKT attempt. But I was pushing the limits now, feeling more like a single frayed nerve end than a complete human.

Old Settlers Trail, while long and devoid of any jaw-dropping vistas or spectacular natural features, is filled with whispers of a bygone era—old stone walls, chimneys, and relics such as enameled bowls and cast-iron pots dotted the 16-mile trail. It was a walk through history—but I was not in the mood to reflect on any of it.

We started our route one hour earlier than normal, despite having just returned from the three most grueling days we'd experienced so far. Our plan was to power through Ramsey Cascades Trail, drive to Cosby to start our second route that ended on Old Settlers Trail, before returning to Buckberry Lodge as early as possible. The following day was one of our "red" days and we'd need to get all the sleep we could before tackling it.

Lane, while planning our routes, color coded them into three categories: green signified routes which were thirty miles or fewer, yellow for thirty to thirty-four mile routes, and red days were anything over thirty-five miles. It was a generalized overview of how demanding the day might be, and we knew better than to assume a green day would always be easier. Elevation gain and loss, weather, water crossings, and especially our bodies' response to the demands we were placing on them, all played into how we'd feel by the end.

Old Settlers was a perfect testament to this, with its constant roller coaster style of elevation loss and gain. I would have much rather climbed a mountain for several miles at a time, versus feeling my legs protest with the constant fluctuation.

I shouldn't have complained—Chris was fighting a far more serious battle against spider webs strung across the trail. Every few minutes, he'd stop abruptly to use his hiking pole to pull the web down before he walked through it.

Occasionally, he'd miss one and find the web on his body, usually somewhere near his face. More often than not, the spider was still attached to the web, making its way onto his face. Chris' trail name, "Pacer," was earned from thousands of miles proving himself as a consistent pacing lead, and he almost always walked ahead of me. I was especially grateful for this during the spider web encounters, knowing my reaction to the spiders on my body would be far more dramatic. But Chris, ever cool headed and compassionate, removed the spider carefully, sending it on its merry way to build another masterpiece.

He missed one spider though, and it slipped down his shirt. "Ouch!" he exclaimed abruptly as the spider took revenge on someone destroying its carefully woven insect net. Or perhaps the spider overheard us talking about the massive quantity of food we would eat that evening when we got off trail—a favorite topic of discussion each day—and was inspired to do the same.

Chris' body reacted to the spider's venom soon after, and he developed a small angry lesion that caused some discomfort. "At least you can't get hookworms from it," I said in jest. Even so, I hoped it wouldn't cause any issues for him later.

Towards the last few miles of the trail, we came across the only two people we would encounter on trail that day—two backpackers heading in the opposite direction. Finally, someone to break through the webs before Chris! We had encountered an abundance of spiders, but Old Settlers Trail is better known for its abundance of copperheads, one of the two venomous species of snakes in the park.

But neither Chris nor I had ever seen one while hiking here or anywhere else in the park. Our spouses, however, had trained their eyes to catch the most camouflaged of them. I chuckled at the thought of how many we were probably passing by and missing as the spiders distracted us, relieved that we weren't noticing them.

That evening, when we returned to the lodge, we discovered a bounty of homemade treats—granola, muffins, cookies, and candy—waiting for us. Kristen Mosley, a fellow Smokies lover and busy mom, had driven from Kentucky to hand deliver them to the lodge. We had never met Kristen, but Jamie had hiked with her before. I considered her a friend, despite only having interacted through social media with her. Unbeknownst to Kristen, she had served as a source of inspiration for me through our training.

After her three children were born, Kristen struggled with maintaining a healthy lifestyle and losing the weight she had gained with her pregnancies; however, she eventually took charge, set goals for herself, and wrestled her health back with hard work and determination.

The biggest challenge of the day was refraining from gorging on everything she brought. But I wanted to savor it and bring it with me in the following days, knowing I'd think of Kristen, inspired by her strength, as I munched away.

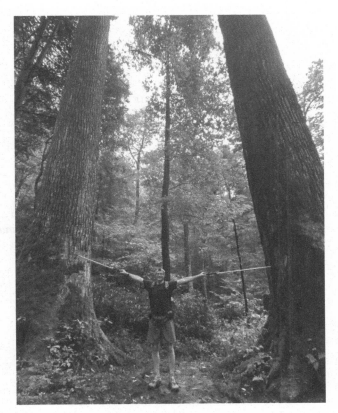

DAY 11: Above, Chris on Ramsay Cascades Trail. Below, Nancy hugs one of the enormous tulip poplars on the trail.

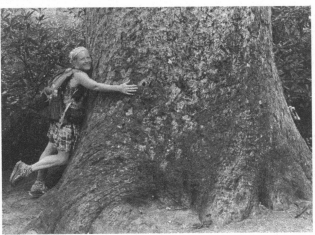

CHAPTER THIRTEEN

Highs and Lows

One of the first things that a young person must internalize, deep down in the blood and bones, is the understanding that although he may encounter many defeats, he must not be defeated.

—MAYA ANGELOU

Day 12—35.4 miles
(6825' gain, 7283' loss)

Over the summer, Chris and I hiked as many of our FKT routes as we could. We assumed it would play to our advantage, testing the direction of them and having a general idea of how long they would take to hike. The biggest benefit, however, was putting more miles and elevation change under our feet.

We practiced this day's route towards the end of our training, and it was where I had fallen and torn a ligament from my thumb. Although it was a random fall that could have happened on any trail (and preferably on one with more bragging rights), I found myself nervous about hiking it again.

The day started optimistically when we forewent making our breakfasts before leaving Buckberry Lodge to treat ourselves to the gluttonous, calorie-rich carbs and fats of a breakfast from McDonald's. It would require a slightly later start since we'd need to wait for the store to open. The extra sleep would be a perk, except that we were facing thirty-five miles of tough hiking plus the shuttle setup with both of our cars. But Chris convinced me that McGriddles were the end all be all of fast food breakfast menus, and we agreed that nutritionally challenged, but emotionally satisfying calories, were worth hiking in the dark for later that evening.

Our mouths were watering by the time we reached the parking lot, but no one answered my repeated, "Hello? Is anyone there?" in the drive thru line. The pandemic had altered many things, including the operating hours of local restaurants. Kristen's granola quickly became the highlight of my day, providing me with a substitute breakfast. Chris, however, had his heart set on that McGriddle, and I could sense his disappointment at missing out on it.

We were in slightly better spirits when we reached the trailhead, and it was easy to work out any lingering frustrations as we climbed Snake Den Ridge Trail. Hiking it reminded us of a group of young backpackers we had met on the trail during our training hike.

As we approached the group, we heard one call out to us, "Is somebody there? How much further is it to the top?" They were ascending Snake Den, hoping to reach campsite 29 on Maddron Bald Trail by dark, but they still had a few miles to go. From the looks of them sprawled out on the trail with enough heavy gear to test the limits of even the strongest hikers, they'd be lucky to make it to the campsite by the next day, much less by dark.

We shared some of our electrolyte tablets with them, knowing their bodies would benefit from the replacement of what they had assuredly lost on the long climb. It was troubling to see them dressed in cotton clothing and lightweight sneakers, outfitted more for fashion than hiking in the Smokies.

Ironically, the extra backpacking gear that was contributing to their fatigue reassured us about their predicament. Day hikers were typically at more risk since many of them neglected to bring what they needed to endure a night in the woods. In a different season than summer, however, we would have been more concerned and tried to convince them to hike out with us. The margin for error was less forgiving in colder seasons.

Later that morning, lost in my thoughts as we descended Camel Gap Trail, I heard a loud noise approaching quickly overhead. The sound reverberated through the mountains and I had a hard time discerning the direction it was coming from. Instinctively, I wanted to seek shelter as fear and adrenaline surged through my body. I ducked and covered my head, flabbergasted that Chris wasn't doing the same. And then it was over and gone as quickly as it approached.

"What the hell was that, and did you think we were about to die?" I asked Chris, wide eyed and shocked. Chris laughed heartily as he replied, "No, those were just F-16s flying over, probably out training." He grew quite familiar with the powerful sound of an afterburner during his career in the United States Air Force.

"Well, good grief, it scared me half to death. I thought with all the turmoil in the world right now someone was attacking our country and we were about to see the end right here during the FKT."

My nerves settled down after the F-16 scare. In theory, I should be more comfortable with supersonic aircraft, since aviation and courage ran thick in my lineage. My maternal grandfather, a consummate Southern gentleman, was a respected World War II pilot who nearly lost his life when he had to bail from his B-24 bomber dangerously close to the earth. He successfully landed with his parachute in a field of peas, but he wasn't sure if they were English or French peas. The farmer, understandably wary of him, circled him with a pitchfork in hand. It was shortly after the D-Day invasion, and they expected a counter invasion from the Germans. Years later, when he would tell the story, my mom or aunt would respond by saying, "Papa, the minute you opened your mouth, he knew you weren't a German!"

He later became the actual poster child for Delta Airlines as a captain on the L-1011—his good looks and warm personality placing him in many ads for the company, alongside my grandmother whom he met on a flight. She was one of the airline's first stewardesses, as they were called then.

My paternal grandfather had an equally illustrious career in aviation, starting as a barnstormer with my grandmother selling food and drinks to their customers in a field below. He eventually became a colonel in the United States Air Force, flying every single plane the branch used.

Working as a flight instructor and pilot for Delta Airlines, my father had long surpassed 20,000 hours of flight time. And my brother was following in his footsteps. The two of them even flew and instructed in aerobatic planes. I was half convinced my family descended from birds instead of primates.

Flying, however, terrified me. My one and only flight lesson from my dad when I was a teenager spurred the fear. Shortly after we took off, the roar of the single-engine Cessna sputtered briefly. I had heard my father swear countless times throughout my life—he had a mouth like a proverbial sailor. But the word "shit" carried a worried edge in the seconds it took for the engine to recover its successful ascent into the air. He later told me the incident happened at the worst possible time, but I knew that if anyone could land a plane successfully in an emergency, it was my dad. After all, he had already proven it when he survived a mid-air collision (through no fault of his). But the incident immediately squelched my curiosity about flying.

Fear had been my constant companion throughout my young life, and this episode only heightened it. It relieved my mom when I came home and told her I wasn't interested in learning to fly anymore. She knew I was a poor candidate for the skills, given my inherent anxiety about the dangers of the world and my insecure manner of responding to them. I suppose my dad did too, but he knew the value of me figuring it out for myself.

In college, a friend introduced me to hiking and backpacking, and I was instantly hooked. Fear be damned, I headed out on a hiking trail every chance I got. There was never a question in my anxious mind that bad things could happen in the woods to hikers who didn't take necessary precautions and learn the requisite skills. But my fears benefitted me since they prompted me to learn the risks and how to mitigate them.

It was an empowering discovery—to forge bravely into the new-to-me world of the wilderness, which was filled with things that scared me. But it also filled me with a newfound courage, inspired by the unparalleled rewards that surrounded me there. While the epic mountain vistas, birdsong, melodic streams, and the lush forest were a feast for my senses, the restorative peace I gained from the meditative act of walking in the woods was food for my soul. I didn't believe in love at first sight until I set foot on a trail in the North Georgia mountains.

As the day wore on in the Smokies however, I was feeling less bold and enamored with the natural world. The climb on Gunter Fork Trail was grueling, as it always was, courtesy of frequent stretches of severely eroded trail, enormous deadfalls lying across it, and an overgrowth of brambles. Unlike trails that began near the park's roads, the interior trails were less frequently maintained. Gunter Fork was steep with multiple wide, and potentially dangerous, creek crossings. The water was low but our slow pace ascending the trail dragged me down mentally.

My mood improved when we encountered a group of retired friends who were backpacking for several days together. Their enthusiasm for life was off the charts, and they peppered us with questions when we told them about our FKT attempt. We needed to keep an efficient pace, but it was hard to tear ourselves away from their good energy and infectious optimism. These friends were genuinely engaged in living fully, for no other reason than the sheer pleasure of being alive.

"I want to be them when I grow up!" I told Chris after we finally parted ways with the hikers. We both agreed to hold each other accountable for staying youthful and adventurous, no matter what age we were lucky enough to reach.

We continued on towards the Appalachian Trail by one of our mutually favorite trails in the entire park, Balsam Mountain Trail. The high elevation spruce-fir forest never ceased to enchant and impress. I half expected to encounter fairies and gnomes every time I traversed it. Thick fog surrounded us on the ridge, which made it even more mystical.

We reached the Appalachian Trail and veered north, skirting Mount Guyot's base, the second tallest peak in the Smokies. When we reached the spot where I had fallen and torn my thumb ligament, the trail was still as gentle and unassuming as it was the day I fell.

The incident was a reminder that trail conditions don't have to be dangerous for accidents to happen in the backcountry. Gunter Fork Trail was a far more likely spot for me to fall and get injured. But I was especially attentive while we hiked it to avoid an accident, unlike this stretch of trail where I let my guard down.

My injury underscored the importance of being adequately prepared on every single hike, to mitigate any unexpected mishaps. Yet so many hikers I encountered through search and rescue operations failed to grasp this basic tenet and ended up in far more troubling predicaments than necessary.

We passed by an empty campsite 29 on Maddron Bald Trail. I wondered how the new backpackers we met over the summer heading towards it had fared. Weariness was gaining on me every second, and I imagined I felt similar to the way they did when we found them sprawled out on Snake Den Trail, trying to reach this campsite before dark.

Short of stopping to filter water or change from our soaked socks into dry ones, Chris and I usually hiked without taking breaks. Our hip belt and shoulder pockets were stuffed with snacks to munch on while we walked, and our water bottles were easily accessed in the side pockets of our backpacks. Cognizant of the ticking clock, we knew the fewer breaks we took during the day translated into more rest at night. But by the time we finished hiking the short Albright Grove Trail, I was irritable and craving time off my feet like a thru hiker craves ice cream on a hot summer day. I typically became quiet during these times, not wanting to burden Chris with my sour mood since he was just as tired as I was, but not complaining.

I stopped to relieve my bladder. My leg had vastly improved, but peeing still required a contorted squat to maintain my balance on the injured leg—my quivering quadriceps protesting the entire time. Usually I laughed at myself during these attempts, despite the pain, while trying to avoid falling or peeing on myself—something I wasn't always successful with on either count. But even humor wasn't helping my mood at that moment.

"We're not even halfway finished with this attempt and you're falling apart at the end of most days. Snap out of this pessimistic crap or you're never going to make it to the end, Nancy," I growled to myself while speeding down the trail to catch back up with Chris. I knew my emotions were stemming from cumulative sleep deprivation. Acknowledging the source of my stress often made me feel better, but I was too far down the rabbit hole of perceived despair that evening. The only thing that would reset my emotions was sleep. Knowing that sleep would be short during the upcoming night frustrated me even more.

While I hiked in momentary solitude, my eye glimpsed a flash of color. I looked down as I was stepping over a heart-shaped rock covered in verdant green moss. I had seen similar shaped rocks every day, but none as beautiful as this one. "A love note from Mama," I said aloud while pausing for a moment to study it.

She would have followed our FKT attempt like a fervent football fan tracks a favorite team heading toward the Super Bowl. And she'd have cheered us on every step of the way, wanting us to succeed with our goal. But she'd want me to learn and grow from the experience most of all. "Win, lose, no matter," she reminded me and my four siblings frequently—a line borrowed from one of our favorite child-hood movies, *Karate Kid*. She'd also remind me that life can change in a blink, and you'd best get on with living while you still can.

Instead of the thoughts lightening my mood, it sent me to a darker place. She was who I wanted to call at the end of this route, knowing that she'd say the perfect words to snap me out of my funk. We talked nearly every day when she was alive. One of the hardest adjustments I went through after she died was instinctively picking up the phone to call her and then remembering I couldn't. Like everything revolving around grief, time was the only thing that helped break the habit—and time takes time.

I finally caught up to Chris and exclaimed, "I am so over this day and ready to be done!" My feet were sloppy from fatigue and I accidentally kicked some rocks which skidded down the trail ahead of me. They were the only noise that filled the silence between us. By now, Chris was attuned to when I needed wordless space instead of a joke to perk me up.

We reached the car long after dark. I couldn't peel my shoes off fast enough as I hobbled to the passenger side of the car. The simple pleasure of sitting down immediately squashed my foul mood. Lifting my feet off the earth was all I needed to erase the memory of my pain.

As we drove back towards Cosby to retrieve my car, I started a livestream video on Facebook with my phone—something we did most days during the attempt to update our followers on our progress and share our "rose and thorn," the high and low points of our day. We hoped they would donate to our fundraiser if our efforts inspired them, especially when they heard the mileage we were covering each day in the name of a cause.

We were still wearing our headlamps as we drove, and we set them to the red light mode so people could see our faces. Almost as soon as we started the video, I was overcome by an intense fit of the giggles.

Maybe it stemmed from looking like ghouls with the shadows cast on our faces by the red glow of our headlamps. Or perhaps it was when I started retelling the story of the F-16's flying over us, fearing we were being attacked while Chris calmly explained to our audience, "Nope, those were our guys." What likely influenced it the most was the incredibly slow and misplaced utility truck we encountered ahead of us, painting fresh yellow lines on the rural road in the dark of night. Chris said nothing about the obscure sighting as I fought to question what we were witnessing through tears of laughter streaming down my face.

Whatever it was, our audience surely thought I was losing my mind, or that I ended each day by numbing my pain with illegal drugs. I didn't care what anyone thought, because the laughter completely refueled my tank and left me craving another long day in the Smokies. It really is the best medicine.

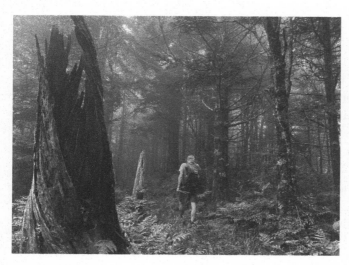

**DAY 12:
Balsam
Mountain
Trail.**

CHAPTER FOURTEEN

Mind Over Mountain

I felt my lungs inflate with the onrush of scenery—
air, mountains, trees, people. I thought, 'This is what it is to be happy.'

—SYLVIA PLATH

Day 13—28.6 miles
(6491' gain. 6206' loss)

During the night, I woke up completely drenched in sweat—so much so that in my sleepy stupor, I questioned if I had crawled into bed after my bath without drying off—only minutes passing rather than hours. I changed into fresh pajamas and moved to the other side of the bed since the sheets were also wet. The evaporative cooling effect of my sweat had done its job of cooling my body down, and I shivered under the covers while trying to fall asleep again.

I hadn't experienced a night sweat since Paige was an infant when my hormones were recalibrating after the hard work of growing another human in my womb. I could only imagine the toll this endeavor was taking on my body as it inched closer to a menopausal state, and I wondered if such episodes would continue in the nights to come.

After the brief night's rest, I expected to wake up even more exhausted. Instead, I felt refreshed, as if the release of sweat had somehow flushed the impurities from my body.

We started the day with a gentle ascent up Lower Mount Cammerer Trail—a welcome change compared to the previous day's initial ascent on Snake Den Ridge Trail. We were both in good spirits after such little sleep the night before. Since we only had to cover about twenty-nine miles, we were optimistic that we might actually get closer to six hours of sleep that night compared to the five hours we normally logged.

This was easy to predict on paper while looking at an elevation profile, but often much harder to execute on legs that were doing the hard work of climbing and descending mountains day after day. The strength I started the day with was a gift, and I promised myself to cling to it as the miles passed.

When we reached the Appalachian Trail (AT), we headed north to Davenport Gap. Each time our feet hit the AT, I wondered about the memories it conjured up for Chris from his thru hike in 2014.

I barely recognized Chris when he showed me his summit photo on Mount Katahdin, the trail's northern terminus, with a full beard covering his gaunt face. Long beards and lean physiques were both common characteristics of men thru hikers who had walked nearly 2,200 miles to reach that spot. I treasured his stories about his "tramily," (trail family) and the bond they shared with the common goal of reaching the end, something only about twenty-five percent of prospective thru hikers ever achieved. Once my kids flew the nest in a few years, I dreamed of thru hiking long trails. Living vicariously through Chris' adventures made me even more excited about the prospect.

Chris shared many tales of his tramily's grit, hiking through multiple days of relentless rain and enduring the treacherous and steep terrain of the White Mountains. But his favorite story was a bizarre one, possibly a first among thru hikers: during his 5-month hike, he never dug a cat hole to poop in the woods. He always used a privy at a shelter or waited until the next town stop before doing his business. One time he even waited four days to reach a town since there were no privies between a stretch of East Tennessee and Damascus, Virginia. He confessed that, "It got serious and I remember wondering why I was doing it to myself." He loved sharing this comical story of endurance, and I loved telling him how much the feat simultaneously repulsed and impressed me.

Besides juvenile challenges thru hikers invent to combat the inevitable monotony of walking through the "green tunnel" of the Appalachian Trail, it was also apparent how much Chris learned about himself. A self-professed workaholic, it was a bold step for him to leave a career that afforded him many material luxuries while also depleting his spirit. He regained his sense of purpose on the Appalachian Trail. Even though he took on a consulting job in the defense industry after his hike ended, he never allowed himself to reach the low point he experienced before setting out. The hike fueled his desire to spend more time in the natural world on foot, prompting his eventual thru hike of the Pacific Crest Trail in 2019.

At Davenport Gap, we sat on the side of the road and waited for Rob, a good samaritan, who offered to shuttle us 1.5 miles down to the Chestnut Branch Trailhead. Rob showed up with even more trail magic — Fanta sodas. I wasn't sure which I enjoyed more, being off my feet for a few minutes or the soda.

Meanwhile, close to where Rob shuttled us to Chestnut Branch, my search and rescue team was taking part in an operation on Big Creek Trail. The day before, a family was recreating at Midnight Hole—a popular spot on the rushing creek where people swam, often jumping off an enormous boulder into the deep pool of water below. Later, we would hear that dive crews found one of the family member's body in eighteen feet of water. The Smokies had claimed yet another life from drowning, the third most common cause of death in the park behind motor vehicle accidents and airplane crashes.

After the steep climb back up to the Appalachian Trail, we continued climbing until we reached the spur trail to Mount Cammerer, site of the iconic octagonal-shaped stone lookout tower built in the late 1930s by laborers and the Civilian Conservation Corps. The day was warm, but we wisely saved part of our Fanta to enjoy while we noshed on a quick snack at the tower.

Each day, we took a photo to represent the number of days we'd been hiking since starting the FKT attempt. Usually, this was as simple as holding up our fingers to represent the number of days we had been hiking. Feeling silly though, we posed as disgruntled, rebellious

13-year-old teenagers to represent our thirteenth day. We both conjured up our best scowls while I held up one solitary middle finger and Chris held up three at a sideways angle—a modified gangster gesture. After the events of the previous four days, it was a welcome change to tap into frivolity rather than fortitude.

Adding to the lighthearted vibe of the day, we later met a trio of local men at Low Gap who dubbed themselves "The Three Amigos." They had been hiking together for decades, and they didn't take life too seriously, at least not while they were on trail together. They reminded me of the backpackers we met the day before, and it was tough tearing ourselves away from their humorous attitude.

During our conversation with the Amigos, we learned one of them had unknowingly lost the glasses hanging from his neck as they ascended Low Gap Trail from the Big Creek drainage. Since we were about to descend and then double back on the stretch of trail he lost them on, we'd have two chances to find them. An impromptu and lighthearted search and rescue effort would be an entertaining way to pass the next few miles.

We found the glasses in short order, and I squealed when we spotted them, jumping up and down with excitement. Even the smallest victories on trail could feel like winning the lottery, especially when it involved paying it forward to our fellow hikers. Jamie would later meet up with and return the glasses to the Amigo who lost them. In exchange, he handed over a generous donation to our fundraiser. There is a common saying amongst hikers that "the trail provides," and it provided in multiple ways that day.

We ended our route on Cosby Horse Trail in the fading light, and I made good on my promise to not cave into self-defeating thoughts like I had the day prior. It was easy on a day like this one. More than any previous day of our FKT attempt, it reminded me of an everyday hike where I had no agenda other than emerging from the woods safely while enjoying myself along the way.

Later that night, back at Buckberry Lodge, I undressed and stood in front of the bathroom mirror while the tub filled with warm water and Epsom salts. At first all I noticed were the usual middle-aged souvenirs of nearly five decades of life—skin tags and sun spots that cropped up like weeds, grey hair stemming from a long overdue visit to my hairdresser, and a network of fine lines continually laying down more tracks on my face. But there was also an undeniable shift taking place in my body. Abdominal muscles that I hadn't seen since my youth were resurfacing. My thighs, while still dimpled with cellulite, were taking on a more sculpted, athletic appearance. My body was becoming a hiking machine, capable of churning out mile after long mile without debilitating fatigue.

I had never considered myself capable of achieving anything more than a participation medal, if I even had the courage to try a sport as a child. It plagued me with insecurities leading into the FKT attempt. Chris, a natural athlete his entire life, had unsurprisingly proven himself a strong distance hiker over and over. My list of long distance hiking achievements amounted to ten days of hiking the Tahoe Rim and Wonderland Trails on vacation.

I knew better than to assume one good day on trail would parlay into the rest of our attempt being just as "easy." But barring any unforeseen injuries or worsening of my pulled quadriceps muscle, the only limitation that could stand in my way was my mental fortitude. "We've got this," I whispered to the athlete smiling back at me in the mirror.

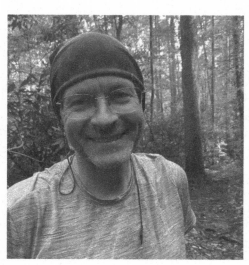

DAY 33: Chris tries out the pair of glasses found for one of The Three Amigos.

CHAPTER FIFTEEN

Rainy Day Blues

"It's a dangerous business, Frodo, going out your door.
You step onto the road, and if you don't keep your feet, there's no knowing
where you might be swept off to."

—J.R.R.TOLKIEN, *THE LORD OF THE RINGS*

Day 14—33.8 miles
(5158' gain, 8075' loss)

"Something's wrong with the women's bathroom door and I can't open it." We were at Newfound Gap with a few miles under our feet after Jamie had dropped us off at Road Prong Trailhead earlier that morning. Passing a bathroom along our route was a luxury I never turned down, especially in cold, rainy weather.

Chris tugged on the door harder than I had, and it opened just enough to discover the problem—it was being held shut internally by a bungee cord. The skunky smell of marijuana wafted by us, and that's when we knew the park's staff had nothing to do with the bathroom closure. Someone was sleeping in it—probably backpackers who wanted to get out of the rain.

It annoyed me that someone could be so inconsiderate of others and park property, but sadly, it was a worsening trend. Since the pandemic started, litter, especially face masks, degraded the trails in certain places. Parking areas filled quickly, and some visitors disregarded the rules and parked illegally, marring natural areas or risking the safety of others with their cars sticking out in the road. It was infuriating to see a place we deemed sacred ground disrespected by some of its visitors.

Our faith in humanity was restored a few miles later when we stopped at Icewater Spring Shelter at dawn to take a brief break from the relentless rain. The shelter was completely full of backpackers, including the exuberant retired friends we had met two days prior. They were packing up to end their trip at Newfound Gap and taking another backpacker with them, giving him a warm, dry place to wait out the remnants of Hurricane Sally.

A quick peek at the radar on my phone's weather app didn't look encouraging. An enormous blob of color in varying shades filled the screen. The rain wasn't ending anytime soon. We would spend most of our day on the high elevation ridgeline of the AT remain cold, windy, and wet.

There was nothing to do but rip the bandaid off and start hiking. So we carried on, protected as best as we could—a delicate balancing act of sufficient layers to stay dry and warm but not so many that we became soaked in sweat.

The stretch of the Appalachian Trail from Newfound Gap to Cosby Campground, where our route would end, offered some of the best views in the park on clear days. But they were nonexistent in the thick fog. Still, the forest was filled with an ethereal quality that enchanted me.

I never minded hiking in the rain if I could stay comfortable. Over the years, other hikers would question and even laugh at my hiking umbrella; however, I typically got the last laugh when I could stay drier under it, especially when the weather was too warm to wear my rain jacket without sweating profusely. Even the most expensive, breathable rain jacket I owned didn't hold a candle to preserving my sanity like my umbrella. But it was useless in windy conditions since a powerful gust could turn it inside out and likely ruin it. For that reason, it stayed packed away for most of our hike along the blustery ridgeline.

Despite the rain, I was in good spirits—the good vibe from the previous day carried into my outlook for this one. Chris, however, was struggling more than usual. He had less tolerance for the rain than I did, and he was more quiet and reserved as we hiked along, partially from fighting to stay awake.

I always knew when Chris was more tired than usual when he wove down the trail, fighting off the urge to fall asleep. Indeed, it was the perfect rainy day to be snuggled up with a great book by a warm fire, rather than hiking nearly thirty-four miles in the higher elevations of the Smokies.

Our route entailed an out-and-back segment on a section of Hughes Ridge Trail, so we took another opportunity to get out of the rain at Pecks Corner Shelter and eat a snack. As we sat and ate, I was acutely aware of how cold it was outside. Our constant motion warded off the effects of the cool temperature sufficiently, but my body shivered—a signal that it was time to pack up and keep moving.

As the day wore on, the cloud cover and tropical storm fueled rain didn't lift, but Chris' spirits did. We reverted to our chatty selves, laughing and making up stories as we hiked. We always cycled back to humor when things were especially challenging. Over the years, hikers have set many FKT records, but it's hard to imagine that anyone had more fun setting one than Chris and me.

We interspersed our lighthearted banter with more serious discussion of how we might reorder our routes over the next few days, since the existing plan included some of the notorious high-water creek crossings from the park's hiking map. All the rain hitting us as we hiked along the spine of the Smokies would funnel into the drainages below, potentially creating angry torrents of water which might be unsafe to cross, especially if the showers continued into the night.

Chris would always have less aversion and more confidence than I did about creek crossings. This was at least partly attributable to a cold winter's day nearly two years prior.

February 16, 2019

Amid my first 900-miler map of the Smokies, I completed a 2-day route with a MeetUp Group hike. The group didn't want to hike the same route as I did on the first day, so I took off solo and planned to meet them at campsite 70 before dark.

I was on schedule until I encountered a wild hog about fifty yards from me on Jonas Ridge Trail, about a mile and a half before the campsite. He was rooting along the edge of the trail when I saw him—the water from the creek so loud from recent rains that he didn't notice me.

It was my first encounter with a wild hog in the park, and I worried I might startle him, causing him to charge me once he realized I was there. But I also needed to get by him. It was already dusk, and I wanted to get through the upcoming creek crossings before it got darker.

I was intentional in my actions before startling him. I had my bear spray with me, so I pulled it out, removed the safety clip, and had it aimed should he charge me. "Hey piggie!" I yelled at him. He raised his head, startled when he saw me, then took off down the trail, running in the same direction I was hiking. I realized his action only partially resolved the problem when I came across him again a few minutes later, rooting in another spot alongside the trail.

This time he noticed me, but he wasn't as spooked by my presence. He stared at me, his tusks reminding me of the damage he could do. Then he focused his attention on the ground again. "I need to get to camp before dark, so can you keep moving, please?" I yelled at him.

Indifferent, he glanced up but didn't move. I had heard somewhere that wild hogs don't possess great eyesight, so I wondered if making myself look bigger might intimidate him more. I waved my poles above my head wildly, even tapping them together to make noise. Lickety split, he took off down the trail.

This was a pattern that we repeated a couple more times—he would run down the trail and I'd soon catch up to where he stopped, waving my poles and scaring him off. Finally, he bolted off to the side of the trail and up a hill just before I reached an unbridged crossing on Jonas Creek.

All the crossings had been higher along Jonas Creek that day, but this one gave me pause. A quick glance at the picture of the park trail map I kept on my phone, besides the paper topographical map I carried in my backpack, revealed what I feared I'd read—the park listed it as one of the particularly dangerous crossings after heavy rains.

The list didn't lie, and I faced a decision—take my chances and ford the angry, churning creek water by myself or stay put on this side of the river and hunker down, giving the swollen creek more time to drain before crossing it the next morning. Do wild hogs ever attack humans in tents, I wondered? I didn't think so, but using my body as a test case wasn't an appealing option. I also didn't want my waiting friends to worry about me if I didn't arrive at camp.

I found a spot downstream from the trail that seemed more reasonable to cross in the high water, and I decided it was worth a try. If the force was too much when I entered the frigid water, I'd get back on the bank and reassess my options.

To stay as dry as possible, I took off my leggings and tucked the hem of my dress into my underwear. I even debated taking my dress off, in case I took a plunge. But I had plenty of other dry clothes in my pack, so I decided to not waste anymore time since it was getting darker by the minute. I unclipped my hip belt and took my first tentative step off the bank.

"Whoa, that's cold!" I said to no one, except perhaps the wild hog watching the scene from a tucked away spot in the woods, undoubtedly pegging me a fool. The rush of the water pushed at my thighs, but it felt possible to cross safely, so I continued on.

Step by careful step, I made my way across, the water rushing at me so hard that it caused my poles to vibrate when I planted them on rocks for balance. My attempt to keep my dress dry was futile—the water was as high as my hips in spots. The deepest channel was on the far side of the creek, but there were large boulders peeking out from the water that I could grab onto should I need them.

Once I was safely on the other side of the creek, my legs and feet felt like chunks of ice and I could barely feel my feet touching the ground. I still had a couple more water crossings ahead of me, but they weren't as worrisome as what I had just faced. By the time I reached camp where my friends were waiting, I was shivering from the cold winter air.

Lynn, one of my friends at the campsite, was tucked away in the woods to use the bathroom. She emerged shortly after I arrived and told me, "I watched you walk down the trail from where I was squatting. Less than a minute after you passed, a wild hog came running down the trail behind you."

It was hard to conceive that the same wild hog I saw earlier had forded the swollen creek. The campsite looked like someone had come into it with a rototiller, indicating multiple wild hogs in the area. No matter which decision I made that evening, I was going to be surrounded by pesky and invasive pigs. But at least I was safe, dry, and in the company of other people.

That night, as I reflected on the day, I promised myself to never neglect looking at the park trail map's list of dangerous creek crossings again while planning routes. I also promised to never cross one that gave me as much pause as Jonas Creek did that day, especially if I was by myself. I had no interest in adding my life to the ever-growing list of drownings in the park.

🐗   🐗   🐗

It was dark by the time Chris and I reached the bottom of Low Gap Trail. Spent from our extensive discussion about possible reroutes coupled with the day's nasty weather, we ended up hiking down the wrong segment of trail that we needed to complete the network of Cosby campground's confusing labyrinth of foot paths.

Backtracking was never a fun endeavor, but especially at the end of a long day during a speed record attempt. It was a quick detour since we discovered it within a few minutes. Chris was always mindful of his designated role to ensure a legitimate FKT by hiking every step of open trails, no matter how tired he was. I was far more grateful for his attention to this task than I was from the minor inconvenience of a few extra tenths of a mile.

While Chris drove us back to Buckberry Lodge, I researched water levels in other areas of the park. The Gatlinburg area had received far less rain than where we'd been hiking, and we'd be able to keep our routes in the original order. It was the best trail magic we could have received after a long, soggy day.

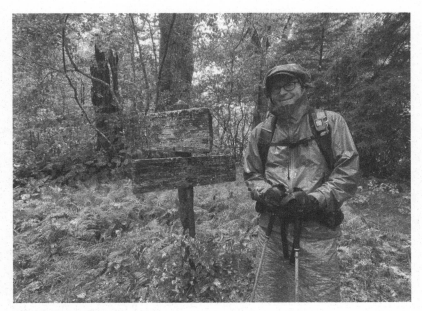

DAY 14: A long, soggy day.

CHAPTER SIXTEEN

Stop Buggin' Me

Repetition will callus your mind.
—DAVID GOGGINS

Day 15—30.2 miles
(4246' gain, 8534' loss)

"Aaaaah! I have another bug in my ear!" We were hiking along Miry Ridge Trail in similar conditions to the first time a bug took up residence in my ear canal, when another insect decided it was worth exploring. Except this one buzzed much louder than the first, which elicited a louder reaction from me in response. Chris, now a reluctant expert at extracting bugs from people's ears in the backcountry, didn't waste any time pulling out Q-tips and his small flashlight. It surprised us to be in this position again, but we knew there was nothing else to do except stop and get it out.

Thankfully, it took little effort, and the bug's life was miraculously spared when it abruptly flew out of my ear and back out into the woods. I had been sleepier than usual prior to the bug incident, but I had no problems staying awake afterward.

We paused briefly at the massive stone fireplace in campsite 71, a remnant of the Bee Gum Civilian Conservation Corps camp, so we could pose for our daily photo. Creating Roman numerals with our hiking poles raised over our heads to look like an "X" and a "V", the fireplace as our backdrop, became one of my favorite photos from the attempt.

The creek crossing on Jonas Creek Trail where I had my winter encounter with a wild hog was hardly recognizable during the low water levels of late summer, even after the previous day's rain. Panther Creek's crossing, another listed on the park trail map as potentially dangerous, was similarly low when we crossed near the end of the route.

Except for the bug flying in my ear, the day was quiet and uneventful. One thing I treasured most about hiking with Chris was the comfortable silence between us. Both introverts, we needed ample time to "hike around in our own heads," as Chris would say.

The silence also eliminated the crutch of Chris' companionship, allowing my fears to take center stage in my mind. This usually created a stream of consciousness centered on "what if's."

What if the new pain in my foot is the beginning of a stress fracture; what if my injury flares up and I can't walk efficiently again; what if someone in my family gets COVID and is really sick...what if, what if, what if. The most constant of these was a deep-rooted fear that I couldn't ever seem to get over—what if I simply wasn't capable of achieving a goal as lofty as the one set out before me?

The incessant loop of anxieties was hard to shake, and it was exponentially more draining than my physical fatigue. Chris' company was far better than the company I kept in my head sometimes. Yet I knew I needed to lean into these insecurities and fears if I ever stood a chance to overcome them.

My "what if's" could become a reality, and some had enormous power to take me off the trail. What mattered the most would be my response to any of those things happening. Yet I wasn't sure how well I would handle it. I knew it would likely send me into a spiral of self loathing if my body failed me. The only thing that gave me solace was to recognize the absurdity of those thoughts, even if I hadn't quite figured out how that would affect my response if it happened.

As for my fear of failing because I wasn't strong enough, I knew the only way to wrestle that one to the ground was to keep putting one foot in front of the other. "It's just walking," I reminded myself *ad infinitum*. But sometimes we need to get out of our own way to move forward.

Jamie was waiting for us at the end, and once again, we ended the day successfully. My tired muscles and joints throbbed in the car on the drive back to Gatlinburg, but the discomfort was a small price to pay to be one day closer to achieving the FKT.

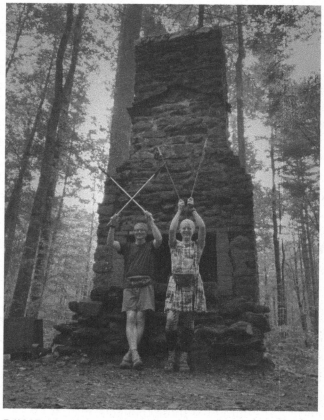

DAY 15: Marking the fifteenth day with Roman numerals.

CHAPTER SEVENTEEN

Family Fun

"Never let the flow of life carry away your dreams."
—WOGENE EAST (MY SON) IN A MOTHER'S DAY CARD
HE MADE FOR ME, AGE 13

Day 16—29.6 miles
(3322' gain, 7704' loss)

I woke with a special incentive to knock our miles out as quickly as possible—my family was coming into town that afternoon. They would travel in our new camper van, visit and have dinner with me at Buckberry Lodge, but stay the night at Elkmont Campground since I started my day so early.

I sought to learn from the experience away from them. At home, I was constantly seeking balance as a wife, mother and professional. The lines were increasingly blurred, with no clear delineation between my various roles. And I obsessed over every decision I made as a parent—was I too strict, too lenient, too this, too that. Our hard work as parents was paying off though—our kids were doing just fine in all the ways that count. But raising them was unequivocally the biggest challenge of my life, and I didn't want to screw it up.

There were parts of my everyday life that I didn't miss at all: monitoring the time my kids were glued to their phones or video games, or the exorbitant time I spent planning, shopping for, and preparing meals for three growing teens and a husband, all while trying to maintain some semblance of a career in veterinary medicine.

I was only working a limited part-time schedule in a small animal hospital before the pandemic hit. I worked enough to justify the expense of keeping my license current, but not enough to stay abreast of the latest changes in medicine. My clients, patients and the staff I worked with were great, but I struggled mightily with constant thoughts of retiring to pursue a different career centered on outdoor education and spending more time in the backcountry.

My exposure to search and rescue operations opened my eyes to how little many people knew about the risks they took when they set out on a trail. Susan Clements' death was the most compelling evidence of how quickly things can turn deadly, and I craved opportunities to put myself in front of hikers and spread the message of safety far and wide. I was quietly using the time during the FKT to assess whether I wanted to return to my career as a veterinarian once it ended.

Hiking stripped life down to the most basic needs and objectives; I simply needed to walk until I reached the end of our day's route, with no one to take care of but myself. Our long routes left me with ample time to think. It was a temporary but a welcome change to the life I had known for over seventeen years since becoming a mother. Still, the separation from my family constantly pulled on my heart strings while we hiked.

Our day started at Clingmans Dome, and within minutes of hiking, a piece of reflective thread from a small bungee cord lying on the ground caught Chris' eye. The week prior, I had accidentally dropped the same thing, but in a different color. I used it to attach my umbrella's stem to my backpack's shoulder strap. It kept my hands free from holding anything other than my poles while I walked. I was bummed about losing this small and inexpensive, yet important piece of gear to help protect me from rain.

On this day's route, Susan Clements was heavy on my mind since we were hiking the segment of the Appalachian Trail where she tragically lost her way and died in September 2018. I couldn't help but think her spirit had a hand in Chris finding the bungee, knowing it would protect me from the elements. It's what a kind and caring person would do for a stranger, and I knew that's what Susan had been.

When we arrived at the shallow saddle near the Goshen Prong Trail turnoff, I paused and looked to my left at the faint depression beside the trail, caused by water runoff. It created a barely perceptible path. It was the general location where I thought Susan likely veered off the trail on the night she got lost—a move that cost her life.

It was a scene I replayed in my mind dozens of times, but it never stopped haunting me—Susan stumbling through the fog and rain in the dark of night, the wind on the ridge cutting through her like a blade as it soaked through her cotton clothing.

By that point, she would have needed to find a sheltered location to protect herself from the brutality of the elements. Dipping off the ridgeline to escape the wind would have been a sound choice for someone who knew where they were and could find their way back to the trail. But in my fabricated scenario, Susan's cognitive function was slipping, and she'd lost some awareness of how dire her situation was. She would have hiked three tough miles on the trail to reach the spot where we stood, probably traveling at a slow pace as darkness fell and the weather deteriorated—plenty of time to reach a more advanced stage of hypothermia. The stage that would lead her to remove her clothing and place herself in a frigid creek. "My mom hated water. She didn't like to swim. But after she had taken articles of clothing off, she had gotten into a little creek," Elizabeth explained to her viewers in one of her YouTube videos.

No one would ever know what really happened and how the scene played out. But no matter how the events unfolded, it became one of the most preventable and unlikely hiker deaths the park has ever seen. All anyone could do now, besides mourn the loss of a human being, was learn from it.

I willed my mind to not linger long on the tragedy. It was easy for me to spiral into a dark place from it, thinking about the "what if's" and how they could have saved Susan. Shortly after, we came across one of our hiking friends, Florence, followed by a group of enthusiastic hikers who were following our speed attempt and wanted to take a photo with us. It was the perfect reset to cheer me up and help me focus on the present again.

After making our way down Goshen Prong Trail, the miles clicked by in the Little River Valley. Our typical pace went up a notch until we reached the aptly named Rough Creek Trail. No matter what time of year it was, the last mile was exceptionally tough and we had to complete it both out and back.

The 2016 wildfires, which started nearby at Chimney Tops, ripped through this area causing massive destruction to the landscape. Only charred, exposed earth and tree snags were left in its wake. Without the shade provided from a tree canopy, brambles took root easily and propagated extensively through their root systems.

The area also became a favorite hangout in summer for black bears who gorged on the berries the brambles provided and left enormous piles of scat along the trail. It was almost impossible to avoid stepping in one, given the challenge of seeing your feet while navigating through the thick brambles.

The dead trees, commonly referred to as "snags," were vulnerable to the wind close to the ridgeline on Sugarland Mountain. They fell across the trail in large numbers and the steep terrain on either side of the trail meant hikers had to find a way through them rather than around them.

For people whittling away at the Smokies 900 Challenge, the end goal was to complete every single mile of open trail in the park. But the secondary goal was to lose as little blood as possible on trails like Rough Creek. However, few hikers escaped without a badge of courage in the shape of a scar—courtesy of either brambles or the fragmented limbs of tree snags—as one fought their way through.

The late summer season had facilitated a slight regression of the brambles overhanging the trail. The dead trees that littered the trail slowed us down significantly during our summer training hikes. Now, they were less intimidating since hikers and resident wildlife had created more obvious places to scramble through them.

After finishing our route, we headed back to the lodge where my family was waiting for me in my room. My kids were unusually shy as I hugged them all close to me. After having been away from them for over two weeks, it brought to light how tall they had become as teenagers.

"I miss you guys so much, but I'll bet this is like a vacation for you, not having me there to police technology time or make you do your chores." My words were an attempt to break the ice and get the conversation flowing with them. What ultimately facilitated the process was allowing them access to the piles of trail snacks I had scattered all over the living room. Gummy bears and Mike and Ike's were just the ticket to loosen their tongues.

We had dinner together, and they stayed much later into the evening than I should have allowed. At home, with everyone's full schedules, we were hardly all together in one room anymore. I knew their visit would provide more strength to me than sleep. I sat on the couch nestled up to Larry, my head resting on his chest while we all talked. The comfortable familiarity of his calm presence was just what I needed to relax and enjoy our brief time together.

Reluctantly, I ushered them out when I started dozing off in Larry's arms. I still needed the physical benefit of sleep to power me through the next day's route, despite how much my family was filling my tank in equally important ways.

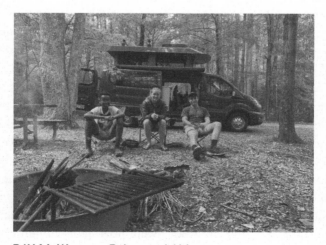

DAY 16: Wogene, Paige, and Aidan at Elkmont Campground.

CHAPTER EIGHTEEN

Stand by Me

If you have ever gone to the woods with me, I must love you very much.
—MARY OLIVER, *HOW I GO TO THE WOODS*

Day 17—33.5 miles
(4079' gain, 8378' loss)

The next morning, invigorated by my family's visit, I woke up alert and ready to hike, despite only getting about five hours of sleep. Our route, while long, had over twice as much elevation loss as gain. I knew my knees would let me know how they felt about things during the 8,000 feet of elevation loss, but a route with only 4,000 feet of climbing felt like an FKT vacation.

While planning our routes, this one brought to light how much distance we'd cover in a day. It started near the center of the park on Sugarland Mountain Trail (off of Clingmans Dome Road) and descended all the way to Little River Road. From there, we would then climb past Laurel Falls and head in a southeasterly direction towards Cades Cove, nearly reaching it before we got off the trail at Schoolhouse Gap.

As we traversed the ridgeline of Sugarland Mountain, the air was cool and the early morning skies were now light enough to see the fog shifting around us. The 2016 fires had scorched this area, but in doing so, had created spectacular views. I loved the contrasting vistas from its high perch—the long ridgeline of Mount Le Conte's summit parallelling us to the right and the distant sounds of the Little River far below to the left. The highs and lows of the park geography felt befitting of our FKT attempt. Within moments I could vacillate between a full spectrum of emotions—believing in my abilities in one breath, then plummeting to the depths of my doubts the next.

But as I watched Chris glide through the fog ahead of me, marveling in the splendor of the 360 degree scenery around me, I was solely content with the gift of our attempt—neutral in my belief or disbelief of what I was trying to achieve. What mattered the most was that I had the honor and privilege to attempt it at all, and with one of the truest friends I'd ever known.

My friendship with Chris was unconventional to some—both of us married to other people, yet completely comfortable with each other while we were isolated in the woods together day after day. We were always cognizant of the marital vows Larry and Jamie entrusted us with honoring—integrity was a vital component of our friendship—but there was never awkwardness or pretense surrounding it. While there was an undeniable bond between Chris and me, it was undoubtedly platonic.

Our spouses both received plenty of curious questions about our friendship, though. It seemed strange and perhaps even inappropriate to some. But I hardly gave our gender differences a second thought anymore, and I often forgot that others might find our companionship odd. These inquires also amused us—every ounce of our energy was being poured into our filthy, stinky, and exhausted bodies successfully completing our goal. A salacious love affair was the furthest thing from either of our minds.

The day passed by with the same familiarity as the days preceding it. By the end, I couldn't believe how long a day could feel when your only aim was to hike over thirty miles and finish before dark. It was a distinct contrast to the hustle and bustle of everyday life, when there were never enough hours to get everything done. Life whizzed by me faster and faster each year as I approached my fifties, so I did my best to interpret the slowness of our days on trails as a gift, too.

Jamie picked us up at Schoolhouse Gap, and we drove back to Gatlinburg with work left to do—pack up all our belongings, including the ridiculous amount of trail food I still hadn't worked my way through. The next morning, we would leave Buckberry Lodge and not return. Instead, Chris and I would leave my car parked at Cades Cove Campground, hike our route, and then ride together to The Hike Inn, a small hotel that catered to hikers, close to Fontana Lake and the Twentymile trail network.

It was our second transitional move around the park and one more big step towards the completion of our attempt. We were well over halfway through our journey. For the first time since we started, I realized that time was flying by, despite the way I felt hour after hour as we hiked.

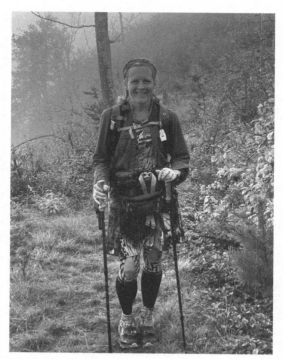

DAY 17: Sugarland Mountain Trail.

CHAPTER NINETEEN

The Thin Place

Hope is the thing with feathers that perches in the soul.
That sings the tunes without the words and never stops at all.

—EMILY DICKINSON

Day 18—27.2 miles
(4865' gain, 4585' loss)

As I was making one last pass through my room at the Buckberry Lodge, I pulled back the sheets on my bed to make sure nothing had gotten tangled up in them. I noticed an envelope with my name written on it. I later discovered that Larry had left it on my pillow the night of my family's visit. In my sleepy stupor each night, I had failed to find it until that moment. It had migrated further down into the bed with my interminable tossing and turning to get comfortable each night.

I had known this handwriting since I was fourteen years old. I had a collection of similar letters spanning the course of thirty-five years in a shoe box back home. Larry had a gift for conveying the depth of his love for me and our relationship in writing. I was nervous to open this one, fearful that it would break my focus and send me into a spell of homesickness. But, of course, I read it, anyway.

He had written a string of affirmations of what he loved most about me, while reminding me of how proud he was of my effort. But there was also a confession of how much he missed me and that he didn't want to be separated for this long, ever again. I was somewhat surprised and also relieved. After nearly twenty years of marriage, I'd expected the time apart would be an appreciated break for him rather than a burden.

My personality in our day-to-day life could be intense and head-strong—qualities that sometimes made me challenging to live with. I was also prone to periodic bouts of melancholy that were nearly impossible to hide or ignore. Larry, in contrast, had an easy going personality. He was nearly always unflappable, despite any challenges that were bearing down on him.

One of the greatest benefits we gave each other in our marriage was time off to pursue our own individual interests without our entire family in tow. Larry usually spent his time on ski or golf trips with his friends. For me, it almost always centered on hiking somewhere.

My multi-day hikes helped me hit the reset button on my emotions, helping me face the challenges of raising children and running our household with less stress. In addition, they provided the space and time to unearth the suppressed lighthearted, carefree version of myself—the one Larry fell in love with so many years ago. It was always a refreshing revelation to discover she still existed, both to me and Larry, upon my return home.

I sat on the side of the bed as I read his letter, wiping away tears of relief that he actually missed me, despite the complexities of my personality. Until that moment, I had needlessly worried. Now, I had all the proof I needed that I'd come home to open arms.

With a spring in my step, we set out on the Little River Trail, starting one of the easiest routes of our entire endeavor. This was the last route we practiced during our training. We had kept a fast pace throughout the entire training hike, ending a year and a half of hard work on a high note, feeling confident about the FKT challenge ahead of us.

After hiking up, then back down Greenbrier Ridge Trail, we started the climb up Lynn Camp Prong Trail, heading towards Miry Ridge. Our conversation tapered off, leaving me to face the thoughts swirling around in my head.

Those thoughts started with the usual topics—obsessing over every tired ache in my body and wondering if it would become more than just a nuisance, followed by mental hiker math to calculate how long it would take us to get to each trail junction and off the trail for the day. Daydreams of what kind of food I was craving for dinner usually followed next. This is when a new conversational thread with Chris usually ensued, when I'd ask him what food he was craving. But instead of waking up our stomachs with conversations of decadent calories this early, I shifted my thoughts to one of my favorite tricks of distraction—silently singing to myself.

Focusing on the recall of lyrics helped steady my mind for an extended period. One specific song often took root more than others and became my earworm for the rest of the day. Here, it was a hymn I had memorized years ago, "For the Beauty of the Earth," after I heard it in my favorite movie rendition of Louisa May Alcott's book, *Little Women*

> "For the beauty of the Earth,
> for the beauty of the skies.
> For the love from which our birth, over
> and around us lies.
> Lord of all to thee we raise,
>   this our hymn of grateful praise.
>
> For the beauty of each hour,
> of the day and of the night.
> Hill and vale and tree and flower, sun
> and moon and stars of light.
> Lord of all to these we raise,
>   this our hymn of grateful praise.
>
> For the joy of human love.
> Brother, sister, parent, child.
> Friends on earth and friends above, for
> all gentle thoughts and mild.
> Lord of all to thee we raise,
>   this our hymn of grateful praise."

Over and over, I sang the verses to myself, the exercise of recall as effortless as breathing once I pulled them free from the cobwebs of my mind. And then, my mother's voice joined mine, softly singing the lyrics with me. I recalled the memory of us sitting together in a movie theatre, watching the scene in *Little Women* together for the first time.

My mind then unlocked a Rolodex of memories, playing them one by one as I flipped through it. But instead of just recalling them like the lyrics to a hymn, I felt as if I was living through them again with her.

I'm six years old and standing beside her as she holds my newborn sister in her arms, shortly after I witnessed her birth—one of my most profound childhood experiences. "How do you spell Molly?" I ask her. "M-o-l-l-y," she answers while gazing down at her contently.

I'm eight years old now, sitting on the boardwalk of a rented beach house in the Florida panhandle. My four younger siblings are with us and we're all studying the pink-orange puffs of cumulus clouds suspended over the Gulf of Mexico. The sun is setting as we point out various animals and other objects in their shapes.

Then I'm fifteen, looking into her worried eyes after I'm caught sneaking out of our home to meet my older boyfriend—his poor life choices influenced by drugs, alcohol, and questionable parenting. I inherited her DNA for believing in the potential for good with every human I encounter. But I'm certain she wishes I'd swap it for a less compassionate approach with some of the company I keep.

Now I'm twenty years old, shivering with her in a tent on a bitterly cold winter night in the mountains of North Carolina along the Appalachian Trail. She has no interest in backpacking, but she has too much interest in my safety as a novice backpacker to watch me go alone. So, she insists on coming with me. We make a quick trip to Walmart to outfit her with some gear, none of it appropriate for the conditions we face. But together we endure and survive.

I'm twenty-eight years old now, facing Larry. We're both standing in front of the altar in the Episcopal church I attended as a child. She's officiating our wedding, just as she did for both my sisters—a perk of having an ordained Episcopal minister as a mom. Her homily strikes all the right tones and her voice cracks as she delivers it. She's elated about who I'm marrying—her tears are those of joy.

Time jumps again and I'm thirty-one. She's embracing me as I labor through a violent contraction with Aidan. "How did you do this with five kids and not want medication?" I wail, tethered to my hospital bed by an IV line. "Because I wasn't induced—this isn't normal labor you're going through," she gently reminds me, validating my consuming pain. Two years later, she's filling my bathtub with more warm water as I labor with Paige, my second child, at home, minus artificial hormones and other medications marring the miraculous experience of my child's birth.

I'm thirty-six now, and I'm the one embracing her. Her ragged sobs shake both of us as I kneel beside her chair in a neurologist's exam room. We've just been told that her recent, unexplained neurological symptoms stem from metastatic lesions riddling her brain tissue. I hold her hand as I drive us home from the neurologist's office, both of us still inconsolable. I wonder how many more days I have left to experience this simple gesture of love between us. And how many oceans I could fill with my tears.

Weeks after she's diagnosed and has started futile treatments that will further rob her of health and vitality, I watch her tenderly deliver the eulogy at her cousin's graveside memorial service after his slow decline and death from cerebral palsy. Single strands of her hair are being carried away, one by one, in the light breeze. I wonder if she notices, but I don't have to wonder if she cares or if the scene of a family member's memorial service torments her.

Soon enough, we'll shop for scarves together to cover her bald head. It won't diminish her beauty or her spirit, though—cancer never stood a chance against that.

Fourteen months after her diagnosis, I'm holding her hand for the last time. She's taking an agonal breath from a temporary bed in my parent's bedroom set up by a local Hospice agency. Her eyes bolt open and her head lurches towards me, my siblings, and our father. And then... she's gone. Just like a strand of her hair being carried away in a light breeze.

And now I'm forty-eight, walking up Lynn Camp Prong Trail with her. I see her beauty in every glimmer of sunlight through the leaves of the trees; I hear her tenacity in the call of a pileated woodpecker nearby; I smell her body in the dank, decomposing leaves beneath my feet. She is no longer hiding in the shadows of the mountains. She's been here all along with me—sometimes I just need to take off my blinders to see her again.

I intentionally increase the distance between Chris and me, knowing he'll worry that something is wrong if he hears my stifled crying. But there's nothing wrong at all. In fact, nothing has ever felt more right.

The ancient pagan Celts and even the early Christians coined the term, "thin place,"—a sacred, ephemeral place on Earth where we are barely separated from the eternal world. Many people associate thin places with locations centered on religion—churches, cemeteries, that sort of thing. I've only experienced them in the natural world, however.

But thin places don't reveal themselves to me at five-star viewpoints, like sweeping mountain vistas or at the base of a majestic waterfall. They're more likely to appear where an unimpressed tourist might give a trail a one-star review. They exist where nothing specific in the natural world has caught my attention, but everything consumes it.

Traditionally, thin places rarely involve an interaction with a lost loved one. They are more of a feeling—a hypnotic, meditative state—rather than a stream of thoughts and memories. But on Lynn Camp Prong that day, those two worlds collided.

I didn't tell Chris about my experience until late in the day when we were walking the last mile of our route. Little River Trail lent itself to us walking side by side. "Today was a really good day," I said, looking over at him, smiling, proceeding to tell him the rest of the story. Chris didn't look back over at me like I just sprouted another head. He knew the mysterious magic of this park, too. We experienced it in different ways, but it was there for both of us, all the same.

Just like when we trained on the route, we finished it in great time. For our eighteenth day picture, we set up my phone to take a shot while we stood in front of an old cottage in Elkmont's historic "Appalachian Club" district. Our pose represented where we were headed as we set out into adulthood. I wore glasses and held a book in my hand, representing the scholar heading off to college. Chris stood in a salute, representing his enlistment into what would become a career in the United States Air Force. We positioned our fingers to represent the number eighteen.

The book I held had become a vital part of my education before attempting the speed record—Jennifer Pharr Davis' *Pursuit of Endurance*. Pharr Davis had set the FKT on the Appalachian Trail in 2011, hiking nearly 2,200 miles in forty-six days. It was an unprecedented FKT to set as a hiker, and the record stood for four years before Scott Jurek bested it by mere hours. Jurek, however, ran to achieve the record, whereas Pharr Davis walked the entire way.

The book helped me understand the mindset of record holders and how they succeeded in their goals. I kept it in my belongings during our hike—a security blanket of sorts, in case I needed a quick pick me up from its words.

After jumping back in the car, pleased at our creativity with the day's photo, we headed out of the park towards North Carolina. We were in good spirits, laughing as we drove "The Tail of the Dragon." The 11-mile stretch of narrow highway with 318 hairpin turns was a magnet for motorcycle and sports car enthusiasts. Most of them were likely enjoying a celebratory beer for having ridden and survived it. Two hours later, we arrived at the Hike Inn, our next base camp.

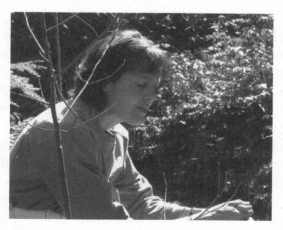

Nancy's mom on Caldwell Fork Trail, 2004.

CHAPTER TWENTY

Evil Creek

No man ever steps in the same river twice, for it's not the same river
and he's not the same man.

—HERACLITUS

Day 19—32.9 miles
(6518' gain, 6535' loss)

We woke in our respective rooms at the modest Hike Inn. Primarily a destination for weary Appalachian Trail thru hikers to take a night off trail before entering the Smokies, the rooms needed little more than a bed, shower, and a dry roof to satisfy.

I scattered my belongings all over the tiny room, and the disorganization knocked the rhythm of my morning off kilter. But it mattered little, because that night we were camping at Cades Cove Campground. My car was waiting on us there, packed with a stash of food, clean dry clothing, and a cot for me to sleep on while Chris slumbered nearby in his tent.

Chris had previously talked me into paying for our rooms at The Hike Inn to store our belongings, rather than load everything back up in his car for one night while we were in Cades Cove. I prided myself on being frugal, but this was not the time to cut corners and make a mistake that cost us the most important currency during an FKT attempt: time.

Our route took us up and over Eagle Creek Trail before we finally arrived in Cades Cove Campground after ten more miles of hiking. Lane, who disliked Eagle Creek's eighteen unbridged water crossings and relentlessly steep pitch near the top of the 9-mile path, nicknamed it "Evil Creek." But before we reached the water crossings, we had a stiff climb on the Appalachian Trail, followed by an infamously steep descent down Lost Cove Trail which was even more evil, by my assessment.

We welcomed the cool morning air on the climb out of Fontana, our tired muscles grateful for any reprieve they could get. The seasons were in transition, morphing from summer into fall. Occasional brightly colored leaves, scattered intermittently on the forest floor, caught my eye as we ascended. Plenty of foliage remained on the deciduous trees towering over us, but the cooler air was reminding them—and us—that fall would herald its arrival soon. I looked down at Fontana Lake far below, smiling at the memories of my family renting pontoon boats each summer—my kids and their cousins being towed on the back in inner tubes, constantly signaling us to increase the speed so they could glide faster across the water.

After making our way across all of Eagle Creek's water crossings, we reached the bend where the trail abruptly steepens, climbing over 1,100 vertical feet in 1.2 miles. Every time I hiked this trail, I challenged myself to not stop more than once during this last mile before reaching the Spence Field Shelter at the top. Sometimes I was successful, but more often than not I stopped multiple times muttering under my breath, "Why do I keep hiking this trail uphill?"

On my prior ascent of this painful segment over the summer, when Chris and I were training, I had a flash of cell reception as we were climbing the steepest parts, and I heard a text come through. It was from Heather "Anish" Anderson, another one of my greatest hiking inspirations. Heather was one of the most accomplished hikers the world had ever seen, setting formidable FKTs on the Pacific Crest Trail and the Appalachian Trail. She also became the first woman to hike the Triple Crown, composed of the Appalachian Trail, Pacific Crest Trail, and the Continental Divide Trail, in a calendar year—a distance just shy of 8,000 miles.

Her message was one of encouragement, and she knew we were in the last stages of training before attempting the FKT. Part of her message read, "The times that seem the hardest are the moments right before the breakthrough. Keep pushing now and remember to rest leading up to the FKT. Sending you all the positive energy!"

I had given Heather and her husband, Adam, a shuttle ride the previous year, picking them up at the end of their thru hike of the Bartram Trail and driving them back to Asheville to their car. I wanted to tell her in person how much of an impact she had on my life—that the courage and strength she wrote about finding in her first book, *Thirst: 2600 Miles to Home,* chronicling her FKT on the Pacific Crest Trail, helped give me the courage to attempt the speed record. The thoughtful gesture by someone I held in such high regard went a long way in powering me up the final, steep mile of Eagle Creek, then and during the FKT when I pulled up her text again for encouragement.

At the Spence Field Shelter, we stopped for a brief break and to take our daily photo. Chris had the idea to stage a scene emulating "American Gothic," the famous folk art painting. Hiking poles replaced the farmer's pitchfork, and it took me several tries to mimic the wife's stern stare at the proper angle. But the shelter made for a perfect backdrop for our backcountry version of this famous work of art.

Later, as we hiked the last mile of our route, we entertained ourselves by reminiscing about our training hike on the same trail. It was a humid, hot day in July and nothing appealed to me more than the thought of an ice cream cone from the Cades Cove Campground store, where we were ending our route and camping that evening.

The warm, humid air slowed our pace though, and we barely made it before they closed. But I was prepared to pick 'em up and put 'em down as fast as I needed to—the promise of ice cream will do that to you. So Chris dialed up our speed a few notches, and we were on our way, arriving with fifteen minutes to spare before they closed.

There would be no ice cream waiting for us during the FKT though—the store closed too early. No matter though, because we found my car waiting for us at Cades Cove Campground with my smorgasbord of food stored inside. We ate a quick dinner, but there wasn't any time for chatting around a campfire and making s'mores. The nostalgic scenes from neighboring campsites would have to suffice.

That night, while sleeping in my minivan on my cot, I woke up famished. As the days wore on, this became a common occurrence in the middle of the night—hiker hunger had officially settled in. I could eat to my heart's content, and it still wasn't enough to satisfy my body's need for calories. This was a luxury with food that I'd never experienced in my life, and I would have enjoyed it thoroughly in less physically demanding times. Food was now an end to a means rather than a hedonistic experience.

With my food at arm's reach beside me on the cot, it was easy enough to fill the bottomless pit of my stomach, even at 2:00 a.m., so I helped myself to chips and chocolate. I fell back asleep with M&Ms in my hand.

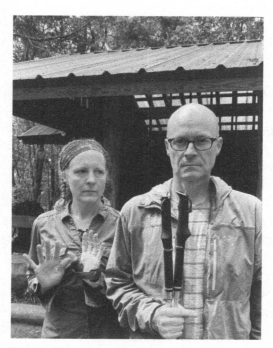

DAY 19: Mimicking "American Gothic" at the **Spence Field Shelter.**

CHAPTER TWENTY-ONE

Stinkin' Jenkins

Almost everything will work again
if you unplug it for a few minutes…including you.

—ANNE LAMOTT

Day 20—32.9 miles
(5309' gain, 5268' loss)

We were up and on the trail by 5:15 a.m., hiking back over the mountain to Chris' car at Fontana Dam. Once again, the morning air was cool, and we made better time than when we had trained on the same route in the heat of summer.

At Russell Field Shelter on the Appalachian Trail, a backpacker informed us of incoming, heavy rain over the next few days. Along the ridgeline, we both had cell reception, so we verified her forecast. A tropical storm would make landfall in Texas soon, and the remnants were heading straight towards the Smokies. Our next few routes kept us away from difficult water crossings, but the thought of heavy downpours didn't sound enticing.

We descended Jenkins Ridge Trail, considered one of the hardest trails in the park by many. No matter which way hikers traveled it, they faced short but steep pitches, leaving them gasping for air by the end. Luckily, the park service addressed the massive overgrowth along the trail the year prior, and we could see our feet most of the way. The downside is that we could also see the how steep the trail was ahead.

We made our way along one of the easiest stretches of pathway in the park afterward—the only open section of Hazel Creek Trail. Most of the length of Hazel Creek Trail was still closed after the bear was found with the hiker's body. We still didn't know if it would reopen before we finished our attempt, but we had a few more days before we needed to figure out when to hike it if it reopened.

We arrived at the Calhoun House in the long uninhabited town site of Proctor, and the front porch beckoned to us like a siren. Lured by the porch the previous summer while training on this route, we had taken an hour-long nap before finishing the final five and a half miles of the hike. A speed record attempt doesn't afford one the same luxury of time, however, so we only stopped for a brief snack break and kept moving towards the finish line.

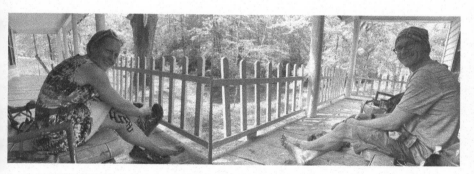

DAY 20: Taking a break on the front porch at the Calhoun House in Proctor.

CHAPTER TWENTY-TWO

Longing on Lakeshore

*I want you to try and remember what it was like to have been very young.
And particularly the days when you were first in love; when you were like
a person sleepwalking, and you didn't quite see the street you were in, and
didn't quite hear everything that was said to you. You're just a little bit
crazy. Will you remember that, please?*

—THORNTON WILDER, *OUR TOWN*

Day 21—33 miles
(4350' gain, 3941' loss)

It was still dark, minus the red glow of our headlamps and the light on
the front of the pontoon boat. Ronnie Parrish, our boat shuttle operator,
knew why we needed the early ride across Fontana Lake, but he probably thought we were half crazy, anyway. Fog enshrouded the lake and
rain pelted our bodies as we made our way slowly across.

We reached the boat ramp at Hazel Creek's inlet and bid our farewells to Ronnie, who wished us luck. Then we set off up the trail
doing what we did best—walking a very long way.

Considered by some to be one of the most lackluster trails in the
park for scenery, Lakeshore Trail winds its way parallel to Fontana Lake
for thirty-five miles before ending at the "Tunnel to Nowhere" near
Bryson City. What it lacked in scenery, it made up for in controversy.

Lakeshore Trail's original intent was to become a road, starting at Fontana Dam and ending at the tunnel. The government abandoned the project when expensive environmental issues were revealed during construction. But the stage was set for tension prior to that, when the Tennessee Valley Authority took possession of 67,800 acres of public and private land to build Fontana Dam, creating Fontana Lake, which displaced many families from their homes. The road was supposed to replace Highway 288 that had become flooded in the lake's creation. A bitter battle between residents of Swain County and the United States Government ensued and continued for decades.

The rain we hiked through felt like a minor problem compared to the residents whose lives were upended by the lake's creation. And with an umbrella over my head, it felt even less significant. Besides, I had trail magic waiting for me at the end of the tunnel. Larry was picking us up at the tunnel and staying with us for the next few days. Several days prior, after my family left Gatlinburg to visit me, Chris and I hatched an idea to elicit Larry's help. But Larry was flying solo with our kids at home, and the plan had many moving parts to secure care for them. Willing and helpful grandparents came to the rescue, and we were all set. It was a surprise and welcome addition to our itinerary.

Our last miles of the day required us to emerge at the parking lot where we were meeting Larry and then turn around and hike the inner loop of the Tunnel Bypass Trail, finally emerging from the Tunnel to Nowhere to end our day. Hiking through the tunnel was always a highlight at the end of a hike. At 365 yards, built under the aptly named Tunnel Ridge, it barely had enough light to walk through without needing to dig our headlamps out of our backpacks. For some, there wasn't enough light, and they experienced vertigo as they passed through—their sense of proprioception altered momentarily. The ceiling dripped with water, which seeped through small cracks, and the walls were lined with graffiti. Voices echoed, and sometimes it was nearly impossible for me to discern if the mouth they came from was standing five or 500 feet away. And on a hot summer's day, the tunnel provided trail magic, acting as a breezeway—the cool air caressing my sweaty body was a magnificent way to end a hike.

Larry arrived early to hike the bypass trail with us. I talked nonstop while munching on my Cheetos—it was hiker happy hour and I wasn't about to forego my favorite snack. I shared every detail about our day, including the only wild hog we saw during our FKT. I hardly noticed how tired I was as we hiked the last miles, too excited by having Larry with us.

After we finished hiking, Larry took a photo of Chris and me with the historic tunnel towering behind us. I felt as strong as the stone walls behind me. The Tunnel to Nowhere signified controversy and frustration to many, despite the $52 million dollar payout Swain County eventually received from the Department of the Interior for not finishing the road. But for me that day, it embodied the passage to an ever-growing confidence in my abilities.

That night at The Hike Inn, Larry sat in the tiny room with me, watching my nightly routine unfold: take a shower, inhale massive amounts of calories, pull out clothes and food and review our route for the next day, along with my favorite task—marking the miles I completed that day on the park $1 trail map.

I always colored the dotted lines denoting the trails with a purple Sharpie marker, in honor of one of my favorite childhood books, *Harold and the Purple Crayon*. There were far fewer trails to highlight now, the purple lines covering over two-thirds of the park's trail network. "I can't believe I've made it this far," I said to Larry. He could though, and it was one of the most endearing things about him—how much he believed in me and supported my mercurial spirit.

The rain fell in sheets all night, pounding loudly on the roof of the inn. Normally, I would have tossed and turned as I fretted about how much it might impact us hiking the following day. But that night, safely cocooned in Larry's embrace, I knew it would be okay. I'd make it through just fine with the extra motivation of knowing he was waiting for me at the end.

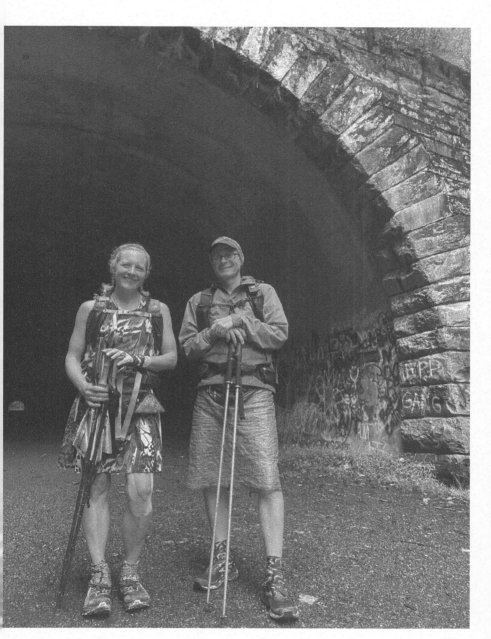

DAY 21: The Tunnel to Nowhere.

CHAPTER TWENTY-THREE

Strong is
the New Skinny

Women are always saying,"We can do anything that men can do."
But men should be saying,"We can do anything that women can do."

—GLORIA STEINEM

Day 22—29.4 miles
(6177' gain, 5551' loss)

"Do you mind if I go ahead of you? I'm pretty sure I'm going to be faster," the backpacker asked us while looking in my direction. We met him as he was emerging from a side trail leading to campsite 113 on the Appalachian Trail, which he had been hiking on for a few days. We didn't tell him why we were hiking, only that we were out for a day hike.

It was an odd request from a backpacker to a day hiker, since the weight we were carrying in our packs was likely less than half of his—not to mention he appeared to have several years on us. I'd never let age define my opinion of someone's abilities, but I normally expected a comment like his from someone younger than me, erroneously sizing me up as decrepit and incapable of keeping pace.

"Sure, yeah, go ahead." Chris answered with a slight tone of amusement in his voice. He looked back at me with a smirk that silently conveyed his thoughts: "Who does this guy think he is?"

About thirty seconds later, hiking behind him at a slower pace than our usual, the man stopped to put his phone away since it was still raining. Chris politely asked, "Mind if we go on by?" Before he could give us an answer, Chris and I hiked past him, up the hill at a faster pace than normal to create more distance between us.

Once we were beyond voice range, we were both eager to talk about the interaction. "Do you think he would have said that if you weren't hiking with me," I asked Chris, suspecting I already knew his answer. "No, unfortunately, I don't think so." This wasn't the first encounter I had with a man who doubted my abilities, and I knew it probably wasn't the last. The same emotions of when I was training for a marathon several years prior surfaced.

One of my long training runs took place on an oppressively muggy morning, and the thick air slowed my pace and resolve. I returned home as quickly as my legs would move to meet a repairman who was scheduled to arrive soon. My doorbell rang with only minutes to spare. "I'm so sorry for the way I look," I told the man, still dripping with sweat, my face flushed beet red. "I'm training for a marathon and my run took longer than expected in this heat." He looked me up and down as I stood before him in my running shorts and tank top and replied, "Huh, you don't really look like a runner."

My mind didn't think quickly enough for an intelligent retort to his insensitive observation, so I brushed it aside and invited him in for the task I had hired him to complete. I knew what a runner should look like to him. My thick thighs, padded with a veneer of visible fat and more similar in girth to tree trunks than pixy sticks, were not part of that image. Yet I was still putting in the same number of arduous miles as someone who fit his concept of a runner, even if I would never be fast enough to stand on a podium and receive an award for winning one.

I was a typical child of the 1980s when "helicopter parenting" wasn't yet a thing. The only playdates my mom organized were between me and my four younger siblings when she needed my help to get dinner on the table. But with nothing more than a Radio Shack TRS-80 computer in our home to tempt me with video games, the

Great Outdoors easily lured me into playing outside from sunup to sundown. I naturally gravitated to the woods and creek behind our house for play. Nature Deficit Disorder, the phrase coined by Richard Louv in his popular book, *Last Child in the Woods*, wasn't an affliction I suffered from. But athleticism wasn't something people ever associated with me, either.

It wasn't until my 40s that I realized I was a stronger than average hiker and enjoyed the challenge of pursuing my limits of endurance. I hadn't found the outer reaches of it yet, which made the quest to find it all the more enticing. Attitudes like this backpacker's only fueled my fire to earn the FKT, if only to prove them wrong.

Later that morning, Chris and I veered off the Appalachian Trail to complete an out-and-back segment to Rich Gap near the summit of Gregory Bald. When we finally arrived at Mollies Ridge Shelter on the Appalachian Trail, we filtered some water before continuing on. While we were completing our tasks, the man we met earlier walked into camp. Despite having hiked an additional four miles, we still reached the shelter before him.

He walked up to us where we were sitting under the side canopy of the shelter, eating a quick snack out of the rain. "I'm embarrassed. You guys were impressive to watch flying up that hill," he said. Chris, while normally humble about our attempt, couldn't resist poking at him a little for my benefit. "Would it make you feel any better if I told you we hiked an additional four miles before getting here?" I sat silent, but smug, interpreting the man's words as "I can't believe this girl is stronger than me." At least he was acknowledging it, and I appreciated his humility.

We left the shelter and continued along the Appalachian Trail, passing the spot where I had been bluff charged by a bear on a solo hike the previous summer. As I rounded a corner on the trail during that hike, I heard a noise to my left and looked up to discover a bear running straight at me and making a noise that sounded eerily similar to Chewbacca from the *Star Wars* movies. I knew I had startled the bear, and I pulled my bear spray out of a sleeve attached to my shoulder strap as fast as I could.

The event unfolded at lightning speed, and I hardly had enough time to process what was happening. The bear stopped several feet short of me and stared straight into my soul. I recalled what a park ranger in Yellowstone once told me—talk to the bear calmly to explain that you're giving it space and heading out for ice cream now, all while slowly backing away.

I knew the ice cream talk was meant to calm me down—and to avoid running, which is the worst thing I could have done. Luckily, the bear bought into my words—or more likely surmised that I wasn't a threat and gave me the gift of living another day. I walked back about a quarter mile and waited for another hiker to come along. I desperately wanted to hike through the area with someone else. But after thirty minutes, I was still waiting and decided enough time had probably passed for the bear to move on. If not, my loud and horrible singing voice would surely drive it away.

Back in the soggy present, as Chris and I were finishing up the same route with exactly zero bear encounters, I saw Larry in the distance, walking towards us on Anthony Creek Trail. I couldn't wait to tell him about my encounter with the backpacker. Throughout the day, my anger had dissipated into humor—perhaps from time passing, but more likely from feeling as if I had just finished stomping chauvinistic mindsets into the ground with each of my powerful steps.

We finished hiking but still had work to do—shuttle my car to the Abrams Creek Trailhead where it would sit for three days before returning to it on the twenty-fifth day of our hike. This meant I needed to get all the food, clothing, and gear that I would need until then and put it in Chris' car. The food supplies I had stockpiled for months leading up to our hike appeared untouched. I had overestimated how much I would eat, despite eating constantly.

CHAPTER TWENTY-FOUR

Water Woes

Love is a maze you can't get out of.

—PAIGE EAST (MY DAUGHTER) IN A VALENTINE SHE MADE, AGE 8

Day 23—33.9 miles
(7039' gain, 7889' loss)

After a restless night's sleep, worrying about the special challenges of the next day's route, I was eager to move when the time finally came. Facing over 7,000 feet of elevation gain and nearly 8,000 feet of loss over the course of thirty-four miles, I admit now that I truly dreaded it. The only thing that gave me solace was knowing I wouldn't have to think about it anymore once it was behind us.

Larry joined us for the first five miles, enjoying his first summit of Gregory Bald. Normally, the bald treated hikers to 360-degree views, but the mountain sat in a cloud that morning, the views completely obscured. Larry bid us farewell and backtracked to the trailhead while Chris and I carried on. Our route took us down the other side of Gregory Bald, losing all the elevation we had gained in our ascent that morning, only to turn around and hike right back up it again.

During our second ascent, it should have excited me that our climbing for the day was nearly over. But we still had fourteen miles to hike, and I was spent. Poor sleep from the previous night—probably only five hours total—coupled with the substantial climbing we'd accomplished, left me feeling more depleted than usual. To make matters worse, the day's route ended with us fording Abrams Creek, which we knew to be swollen after the recent rain.

Lane and another mutual friend and SAR team member, Jackie Kuhn, had spent the previous day shuttling Chris' car from the Twentymile trailhead where we'd left it two days ago, to the Abrams Creek Campground where we'd stay that evening. The endeavor consumed their entire day, with many hours of driving around the park's boundary and then back to Waynesville.

Lane sent us a video of the creek spilling over its shallow banks with the trailhead sign half submerged under water. The water looked like chocolate milk, and I knew it would be deep. The trailhead sign confirmed my hunch. If we reached it and it was impassable, we'd be stuck on the other side, waiting for who knows how long.

Chris felt confident it would drain off enough during the day for us to cross it safely, and I'd learned to put my trust in his opinion with these crossings. But I would fret until I saw it with my own two eyes—I was a master at fretting.

The fourteen miles passed slowly, and despite the easier terrain, my steps were getting sloppy. At one point, I slipped on a slick patch of mud, sending my left hand to catch my fall on the side of the slope. My thumb ligament was healing well, as far as I could tell, but my fresh scar was still tender and I yelped from the momentary pain.

Chris picked up on my anxiety—he always did. To keep my mind busy with something besides the creek crossing, he started a conversation about Thanksgiving traditions in our families. Any conversation between us that revolved around family traditions always became comical. Chris shared his idea to stay in pajamas all day on Thanksgiving one year, preemptively managing the discomfort of a full belly and the unyielding waistline of regular pants. I laughed at the image of him chatting it up around the dinner table with Jamie and her family in all their comfiest sleep clothes.

An eternity still passed before we finally reached Abrams Creek. I looked across it for Larry, hoping he might show up, but he wasn't there. The creek, while still swollen and flooding its banks, didn't look as dangerous as the video Lane had sent us. Chris stepped out into it before I did, to test the depth and force of the water. "It's okay, you're going to be fine crossing it," he said encouragingly.

I exhaled a sigh of relief, agreeing with his assessment. "I agree, I think I'll be okay. Will you just stay close by while I cross?" This was a question I didn't even have to ask. Chris knew how much I dreaded water crossings and when he should stay close by as we forded certain creeks.

The water, chilly and refreshing on my tired feet, was like a backcountry spa experience. I dare say I even enjoyed the crossing. As soon as we reached the other side, Larry came running down the trail. I had texted him earlier to tell him when to look for us on the other side of the creek, in case we ran into any trouble crossing it. I ventured back out into the water and asked Larry to take my picture while I was there. I wanted to soak my throbbing feet in the cool water a short while longer. But more than that, I wanted the picture to remind me how pointless fretting was before I knew all the facts about a situation.

That evening, the stress and fatigue of the day caught up with me again, and I was short with Larry. Every second counted during an FKT attempt, and it was my assumption that he would start heating water for pasta before we arrived. The extra time we spent waiting was time we could be sleeping. I started calculating how little sleep we'd get for the extra time it was taking to boil water.

Larry, conversely, didn't understand how the extra time to boil water could make that much of a difference. When he adorned the pasta with unheated spaghetti sauce and struggled to find eating utensils for us in the van, it didn't help ease the tension that had already grown between us.

In my mind, he had all day to make a simple meal and have it ready for us when we finished hiking. In his mind, he had done plenty of unglamorous heavy lifting back at home, for nearly a month now, to help me pull off the FKT. The least I could do was be grateful he was here to help us, even if dinner took a few extra minutes to make. Marriage is hard, if only for the most trivial of altercations.

The act of executing an FKT was one of the most challenging endeavors I had ever done, but Jamie and Larry had equally difficult roles, if not harder, as our spouses and support team. We were both eternally grateful for the help and support they gave us, and it was unfair to expect them to read our minds. But as is often the case, we take things out on the ones we love the most.

As we laid in our ModVan's pop-up roof bed with Chris below us in the other bed, I quietly thanked him for his support. I was ashamed that I didn't act more grateful for all that he was doing. The head rub he gave me in return, to help me drift off to sleep, was everything I needed in that moment to know we—and I—would be okay.

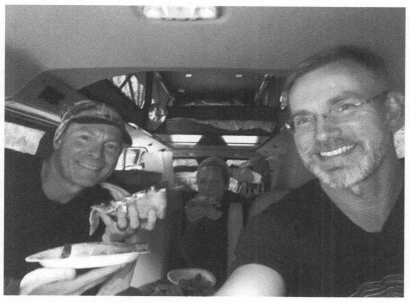

DAY 23: Camping in the camper van.

CHAPTER TWENTY-FIVE

Anxious About Abrams

Solvitur ambulando
(In walking it will be solved)

Day 24—28.7 miles
(3463' gain, 3479' loss)

Before daylight, Chris and I were hiking again, leaving Larry to pack up and head back to our home in Waynesville, North Carolina. I treasured every moment spent with him, even the tense one over lukewarm spaghetti. It was time to refocus on our goal, though. Having Larry in my midst both strengthened and weakened my resolve, and I was feeling the ever stronger tug to return home.

But before I could go home, I still had a minimum of 180 miles to hike over the next five to six days. We were still waiting on the answer to one question before locking in a specific timeline—would the park service reopen the 8.1-mile section of Hazel Creek Trail before we finished our attempt?

No one seemed to know when they might reopen the trail, despite our attempts to find out through various channels; however, based on prior bear attacks on humans in the park, it wasn't unreasonable to think it might stay closed.

One such incident took place in 2016. A bear attacked a 16-year-old boy who was backpacking a 5-day route in the park with his father.

The bear bit the boy in the head while the youth was sleeping in his hammock at campsite 84. Campsite 84 was also, coincidentally, along Hazel Creek Trail.

The teen's father, sleeping in a nearby hammock, awoke to the sounds of his son yelling and rushed to the scene. Miraculously, he fought the bear off of his son. A boat that other nearby campers had used to access the Hazel Creek corridor shuttled them across the lake so they could get to a hospital. The teen survived, thanks to he and his father's quick and appropriate actions. The park made a hard decision and euthanized the bear that had attacked the boy, but when the DNA results were analyzed, the rangers discovered they had euthanized the wrong bear.

While the park service could only do so much to guarantee they had found the correct bear before euthanizing it, these incidents inevitably sparked a lot of controversy, especially on social media. There was still a dangerous bear wandering the area, and now they had to deal with waves of criticism, too. The park closed multiple trails and campsites until they could euthanize the correct bear, which they eventually did.

As far as we knew, the park service was sure they euthanized the correct bear that was found scavenging on the hiker's body during the recent incident. However, motion-sensor trail cameras were now monitoring the activity at campsite 82, to see if any other bears showed up looking for a body that they too may have scavenged on.

We heard that wildlife rangers had checked the cameras twice already, but it was unclear if bears were returning to the campsite regularly. Given the gravity of the situation, especially since there weren't any straightforward answers about whether the hiker's death was related to a predatory attack or not, the park kept it closed a while longer. Better safe than sorry.

If the trail opened at any point before we finished, even if it was during our last foot strike on the last day of hiking the open trails, we'd have to hike that segment of Hazel Creek to claim a legitimate speed record. The scorekeepers for FKTs were a trio of endurance athletes who started a website called "Fastest Known Time" for people to submit and record their accomplishments once they were verified.

There were guidelines on the FKT website to verify speed records: recording and submitting data via GPS tracks and preferably providing additional documentation with time-stamped photos and/or written trip reports. Not everyone followed these guidelines though, placing them in an "unofficial" FKT category, limiting them to making a claim in discussion forums versus having their name recorded on the website's page dedicated to the route. In the eyes of most, including the FKT website's administrative team, athletes needed to provide concrete evidence to back up an FKT if they wanted people to take it seriously.

The website stated that every mile of open trail should be traversed in order to achieve an FKT. If a stretch of trail was closed while someone was attempting the record and it stayed closed for the duration of their attempt, it wasn't necessary to wait until it reopened to hike it and earn an official FKT.

Trail closures occasionally created controversy, though. For instance, if a hundred miles of a long trail, such as the Pacific Crest Trail (PCT), closed for something like wildfires, the playing field between athletes was altered significantly. Unless there was a reroute with a comparable distance, it might void a legitimate FKT attempt. But a few miles difference on a nearly 1,000 mile attempt such as the Smokies 900 didn't matter all that much, at least in the eyes of the FKT organization.

The history of the Smokies 900 FKT had already experienced such discrepancies. During Benny Braden's attempt in 2017, he didn't hike several miles of Sugarland Mountain Trail or Bullhead Trail—a deficit of nearly eleven miles—since they were both closed after the 2016 fires.

But Jeff Woody, the next person to set the record—and the first to provide GPS documentation to verify his success—didn't hike Porters Creek Trail since it was closed for repairs, reducing his mileage by 2.7 miles (which really amounted to 5.4 miles since it's a dead end trail which requires backtracking to the trailhead). Porters Creek Trail was still closed when Chris and I began our attempt, leveling our playing field with Woody's, at least initially.

Furthermore, the Smokies trails weren't laid out linearly like the AT or PCT, and therefore there were overall mileage discrepancies between athletes attempting the Smokies 900 FKT. Competitors had the liberty to create routes that aligned with their capabilities and comfort level. Typically, the more miles someone was willing to hike in a day translated into fewer overall miles they'd hike by the end of their map-marking quest.

In short, the Smokies 900 was inherently more complicated than most approved FKT routes.

Even if Hazel Creek remained closed, it was highly unlikely that a deficit of 8.1 miles would invalidate our FKT submission. We also wouldn't harbor an iota of guilt about it, because it had already derailed Lane's carefully orchestrated plan and added even more mileage to our routes than appeared on the surface.

Since the closed segment of Hazel Creek Trail was deep in the park's interior, it would entail hiking a minimum of twenty-one miles to complete it, roughly adding an extra day to our timeline when we considered car and boat shuttling time. Not to mention, we would finish our FKT in a remote location—at the junction of Hazel Creek and Cold Springs Gap. From the beginning, we looked forward to finishing at the Big Creek trail area, where our family, friends, and supporters could drive in and celebrate our success with us.

Many times during our attempt, I reflected on the sacrifice our families were making in order for us to achieve this goal. They deserved a celebration and recognition as much as we did. Lane, our steadfast trail boss, was also a key player. I wanted him at our finish as much as our families. Our attempt had also attracted a following of supporters, many of whom were asking about our finish date so they could be there with us. It pained me to think of us finishing separately from the presence of all these people who had been just as much a part of our success as we had. For that reason alone, I tried not to think too much about the prospect, even if I knew it could become our reality.

But we had to talk about it. Finding a place to wedge the route in wasn't easy, and we had to strategize and figure out the most logical time to hike it, day by day, depending on when it opened—if it even opened at all. At least it gave us something to talk about for hours on end.

The relatively easy trails of the Cades Cove area of the park allowed us a quicker pace than the previous day, and it countered the stress I was feeling about Hazel Creek. But as we neared the wide and argu-ably most dangerous creek crossing in the entire park, my nerves were on high alert.

I heard the rapids before I could see them below on the trail, and I half jokingly made sure Chris knew how much I loved my life and wanted to keep living it. He assured me he would not let me die and reminded me of the time he was hiking with another friend, who was also nervous about the crossing. At one point, she slipped briefly in the deepest channel and then clung to him the rest of the way, terrified of being swept away forever.

We arrived at Abrams Creek, and it was higher than I'd ever seen it. I wouldn't have dared crossing it by myself. "What do you think?" I asked, tentatively, since I didn't trust my judgement to gauge the safety. "Let me go test it out and see how it feels while you stay here. I'll come back and get you once I find the safest spots for us to walk through." Chris replied confidently.

I wasn't sure if that plan was any better. Aside from worrying about my safety, the last thing I wanted was to watch one of my best friends get swept downstream. Chris, however, had much more expe-rience than me from his months of hiking the PCT, where hikers must frequently cross streams in the Cascades and Sierras that are swollen with snowmelt.

Slowly and methodically, he made his way nearly to the other side of the creek. I held my breath as he traversed the deepest channel, knowing it was the most likely place he might lose his footing. The water rose to his hips, but it didn't appear to be pushing him substan-tially. But it would rise higher on me since I was a half foot shorter than him.

He returned with good news. "You can do this," he said. "I'm going to stay right behind you the entire time and talk you through it, but you're going to be fine." Trust is perhaps the most sacred shared value between friends, and Chris had earned mine long before I stood on the banks of a creek that gave me such pause. So I took a deep breath and unclipped my hip belt in case I slipped and needed to rid my body of the weight quickly to stay afloat. We started across diagonally, side stepping while facing mostly upstream, planting our poles into the rocky and slick creek bed before taking the next careful step.

The water depth rose and fell, sometimes up to my waist while at other times only to my thighs. Chris stayed behind me, just as he promised, calmly talking to me through the spots where I needed extra encouragement to move—fearful that the second I picked up a foot, it would cause me to lose my balance and fall. Before I knew it, we were taking our final successful steps onto the creek's opposite bank.

Chris grinned at me when we were safely on dry land again. "You did it! I didn't want to tell you this until now, but that was actually higher than when I crossed it with Anoria." I laughed and told him I wasn't sure if I felt better or worse knowing that. But ultimately, it empowered me. The water was strong that day, but I was stronger.

We continued on, passing the spot where we encountered a calm but large timber rattlesnake one morning during the previous spring. Chris unknowingly walked by it as it sat coiled up on the side of the trail. "Chris, you just walked right by a rattlesnake!" I exclaimed as soon as I noticed it. We were worried it might not be as docile once the morning air warmed up and other hikers came down the trail, so Chris carefully moved it by scooping it up with his hiking pole. It barely protested, rattling enough to give us a show but not enough for us to worry about a strike.

After the steep climb up Little Bottoms Trail, we descended and finished the route where we began in the wee hours of the morning at Abrams Creek Campground. The smell of campfires and charcoal filled the air, and my hunger took center stage. Jamie was bringing us Carraba's for dinner that night in Townsend, where we'd be sleeping the next two nights at the Tally Ho Inn. I was excited about returning to a land where air conditioning, soft beds, and hot showers were part of my nighttime routine.

We stopped by the grocery store on the way into Townsend and I bought a pint of ice cream. I ate the entire pint, plus my dinner, and I still woke up hungry in the middle of the night.

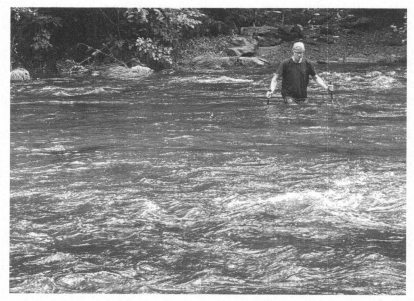

DAY 24: Chris testing the water in Abrams Creek.

CHAPTER TWENTY-SIX

Cleaning Up the Cove

"Finding beauty in a broken world
is creating beauty in the world we find."

—TERRY TEMPEST WILLIAMS

Day 25—29.3 miles
(4592' gain, 5453' loss)

The logistics of our hikes often dictated how late we'd be on the trail, depending on how much time we'd spend shuttling cars or driving to and from trailheads each day. Car time was hard to estimate and even harder to control. Such was the case when we arrived at the Cades Cove gate forty-five minutes before it opened for the day and discovered several cars waiting ahead of us.

We knew we'd have to pack our patience driving through Cades Cove behind throngs of tourists, stopping to ogle every bear, turkey, or coyote they saw. But with the clock ticking, we had little patience to spare. So Chris walked up the line and explained our mission to the couple in front. They were sympathetic to our cause and let us drive ahead of them once the gate opened. We headed to our starting point on Rich Mountain Road, a one-way road centered roughly midway in the cove.

We parked the car and started our route, tackling the Indian Grave-Rich Mountain loop first, then crossing the road higher up to start a long traverse along the park's boundary. Eventually, we descended into the depths of the valley onto Beard Cane Trail, a tough slog in warmer months.

On April 27, 2011, an EF4 tornado ravaged the landscape and left a quarter-mile-wide swath of destruction in its wake. It impacted nearly a mile of Beard Cane Trail. With few remaining trees, the undergrowth of mostly nonnative, low-lying plants took hold and consumed the area. The swampy ground in this part of the park didn't help matters, and traversing Beard Cane was, in short, a mess.

As luck would have it, the park's trail crew had recently maintained the trail. There were still areas of shoe-sucking mud, but at least we could see our feet as we stepped through it.

Despite the easier traverse of Beard Cane, the conditions still slowed our pace. We had to hike Cooper Road Trail too, and it was one of my least favorite trails in the park. It wasn't the toughest trail, but it was still a grind of constant elevation gain and loss, coupled with dry, exposed, hot, and overgrown conditions in late summer.

"After the FKT, I never have to hike Cooper Road again," I said to Chris while wiping copious amounts of sweat from my forehead with my sweaty arm. I often proclaimed this when we hiked trails I didn't enjoy. I knew I'd hike it again—map marking in the Smokies was addicting. But tricking myself into thinking I wouldn't hike it again gave me a sense of control about my current situation. Towards the end of the day, a black bear scurried across the trail ahead of us—proof that every trail in the Smokies bore its rewards if we allowed ourselves to see them, even the ones we professed not to like.

We ended the route by retrieving my car in the Abrams Falls parking area, where I'd left it three days ago. We still had daylight to spare, but it was increasingly clear how short the days were becoming as fall approached. The still and humid air in Cades Cove held onto the remnants of summer though, and the thickening clouds above hinted at incoming precipitation.

I was grateful that it was our last full day in Tennessee and that we were transitioning to the North Carolina side of the park the next morning to finish our quest. We'd spend the bulk of our time in the higher elevations where the air was cooler and the scenery of the northern hardwood and spruce-fir forests enchanted both of us.

But first things first, we needed to pack our cars with the contents of our hotel rooms and wedge in as much sleep as possible. We would spend a brief night in Townsend and begin the next day with a 3:00 a.m. wake-up call to make the two-hour drive across the park to the Balsam area.

On the drive back to Tally Ho Inn, we retrieved Chris' car that we'd left that morning on Rich Mountain Road. Chris took the lead as we drove, and his keen eyes spotted two copperheads on the gravel road, both at risk of being flattened by a car tire from someone less observant or with a vendetta against snakes—an unfortunate reality with some of the park's visitors (despite its illegality). We stopped both times, and Chris coaxed the snakes off the trail with his hiking pole. His altruistic effort noticeably agitated one of them. "He's trying to save your life, big guy," I said to the snake, half amused and half worried that the late hour might retard Chris' reflexes. I put my worries to rest when the snake finally slithered out of sight, and we carried on towards Townsend.

As I scarfed down my dinner, eager to get in bed, I checked the park's website for any updates on Hazel Creek Trail. It was still closed, with no sign of when it might open. Instead of relieving me, it made me feel worse. By now, I was resolved to the idea of hiking it—that wasn't the root of my stress anymore. I only wanted to know if we would need to hike it so we could brainstorm about how to fit it in with the rest of the routes.

Eating junk food in stressful situations was a lifelong habit. But the FKT placed me in a fortuitous position as I pondered the unknowns of Hazel Creek. For the second night in a row, I ate a pint of ice cream after eating my enormous dinner. But unlike my "real life" where I might feel remorse for consuming unhealthy calories to ease my anxiety, I didn't think twice about the indulgence.

CHAPTER TWENTY-SEVEN

Carolina In My Mind

*"I am incapable of conceiving infinity, and yet I do not accept finity.
I want this adventure that is the context of my life to go on without end."*

—SIMONE DE BEAUVOIR, *THE COMING OF AGE*

Day 26—25.1 miles
(6529' gain, 7175' loss)

The drive to North Carolina and Balsam Mountain Road was as demanding as the trails we'd soon hike. Rain and thick fog accompanied us the entire drive of nearly two-and-a-half hours. Chris, who took the lead, had a hard time staying awake, despite the road and weather demanding his attention.

Our hiking would only amount to 25.1 miles, our shortest of the entire FKT, but we would spend five hours driving between four different trailheads and eventually to my home at day's end. Every FKT route comes with its own set of challenges. For ours, one of the biggest was navigating travel logistics and minimizing our time in cars versus on trail. With a park spanning over half a million acres and few internal roads to connect the trails, we often sacrificed sleep or additional hiking miles for commuting.

Chris' foggy state of mind caused him to overshoot the trailhead of Flat Creek Trail and continue down the road to the trailhead at the

134

other end, where he realized what he'd done. His razor sharp attention to detail hardly ever missed a beat—he was clearly struggling. The cumulative effects of sleep deprivation were emerging in both of us.

We eventually positioned our two cars properly at each end of Flat Creek Trail. The trail was a perennial family favorite. It was close to my home and one that my kids hiked with ease when they were younger. The reward of Flat Creek's calm waters, perfect for splashing in and looking for salamanders, coupled with our tradition of searching for the elusive fairies in the expansive fern glades lining the trail, made it an exceptionally fun trail.

But on a dark, rainy morning with a chill in the air and the wind whipping around us, the fairies and salamanders were nowhere to be found. Our mission was to stay focused, to avoid slipping on the slick trail or be taken out by a falling tree. We would also need to be extra vigilant about staying dry, to ward off hypothermia.

Driving between the trailheads chewed up time on the clock, but it also afforded us time to warm up and shovel in calories. But recharging my emotional batteries to music was the best perk.

For months leading up to the FKT attempt, I added to a playlist that I created for motivation while I drove to our arduous training hikes. Songs such as Kanye West's "Jesus Walks," and David Bowie's "Under Pressure" were two of my favorites to energize me. And as corny as it was, Miley Cyrus singing "The Climb," conjured up the image of crossing the last few steps of trail at the end of our FKT. This visioning process was a powerful motivator to reach that point.

But my favorite song on the playlist was Alicia Keyes, "Underdog." I played it on repeat as I sang along with a singing voice that was proportionately horrific in contrast to Keyes' soulful one. Now, as we neared the finish line of our journey, the song's lyrics not only motivated me, but they also validated me.

The FKT was no longer an elusive goal far in the distance that I did not know if I could achieve. I could almost reach out and touch our success. But I suspected we were likely the underdogs in the minds of many people watching our effort, unlike the current FKT holder of the Smokies 900, Jeff Woody, and his long list of impressive athletic achievements.

In July, just two months before our attempt began, Woody, an accomplished ultrarunner from Knoxville who had completed all the Smokies trails eight times, publicly announced he was attempting the Smokies 900 FKT. A quick search on the internet revealed his many accomplishments, including running fifty ultramarathons, one in each state, before he turned fifty years old. Learning about his achievements intimidated me and chipped away at the confidence I'd earned with months of training over thousands of miles.

Jeff succeeded, unsurprisingly, at setting a new and formidable FKT of thirty-three days and eight hours—shaving ten days off the previous one set by Benny Braden. The routes Lane created positioned us to beat Jeff's time, even before we knew of his attempt. However, we lost our comfortable cushion. The race against the tortoise and the hare—the slower hikers versus the faster runner—was still ongoing. But now we had a solid lead that was growing each day.

We made quick work of the 2-mile round trip up Spruce Mountain Trail and back. One of the shortest trails in the park, it rose steadily from the trailhead, ending at the infrequently used campsite at its terminus, perched in a dense spruce-fir forest at 5,500 feet.

We reversed the route and headed downhill, back to our cars, where we continued to Beech Gap Trail. We repeated our pattern of ascending and descending on an out-and-back path. This time, however, our gain and loss amounted to over 3,600 feet over the course of fewer than five miles.

Our fourth and final segment for the day was the most rigorous, covering over fifteen miles with 8,000 feet of collective gain and loss. The rain continued, as did the wind, which forced me to keep my umbrella tucked away and don my rain gear instead.

By the time we reached Hyatt Ridge, the sweat from my exertion while climbing was chilling me beneath my rain gear. It was difficult to move quickly enough to avoid getting cold, given the rooty, rocky conditions of the rain-soaked trail. I was shivering and having trouble holding onto my hiking poles, so I knew hypothermia was creeping up on me. "I'm getting pretty cold and a little worried about it getting worse," I told Chris through my chattering teeth, hoping that by saying the words it might ease some of the anxiety.

Chris knew these were words to take seriously and insisted we stop so I could remove some of my wet clothing. As counterintuitive as removing clothing seemed, it was the only way I stood a chance of getting warmer. Chris walked down the trail to give me some privacy, but it made me nervous to be alone. "What if I can't make my hands work to change clothes and I get even colder?" I thought to myself. I knew how quickly the more serious effects of hypothermia could sneak up on someone, and the last thing I wanted was to force us off the ridge to the warmer air at lower elevations.

I fumbled to unbutton the synthetic shirt I was wearing over my dress. It was damp with sweat and from rain water trickling under the cuffs of my rain jacket's sleeves. My rain skirt was soaked through, and the fabric clung to my bare legs, making me colder, so I removed it next. I intended to remove my dress and bra and replace them with my alpaca fleece hoodie, since it was one of the few dry clothing articles I had left in my pack. The properties of the wool fibers would keep me warmer, even if they were damp, compared to the synthetic clothing I was wearing. I usually wore a pair of running shorts under my dress, so I didn't need to worry about modesty while climbing up, over, and under various obstacles in the trail. If I needed to remove my dress and hike only in the hoodie, the shorts would prove a godsend. Luckily, my dress felt drier than I expected. I pulled the hoodie over it and put my rain jacket on last. The alpaca wool felt like a warm hug around my body, and I knew instantly that I'd warm back up once I started moving.

By the time we started climbing beside Enloe Creek, the rain slowed down to a light drizzle, and the surrounding forest was cloaked in mist and fog. The roar of the creek below overrode my fear of hypothermia with nervousness about the unbridged crossing up ahead. While it was indeed flowing heavier than normal, we could manage it well.

We climbed steadily up the rutted, muddy trail towards our turn-around point at the junction of Hughes Ridge Trail. As we ascended, so did my mood. Despite the poor weather during a long, drawn out day, I would see my family and our beloved dog, Josie, soon. I smiled at the thought of our big, goofy rescue girl with two different colored eyes greeting me, jumping up and down on her two front legs, probably farting simultaneously.

Thoughts of my family made time drag even slower. It would still be hours before we pulled into my driveway, and I needed to stay focused as we descended the same slick trail we'd just climbed. To occupy my mind, I started singing "Tomorrow" from the musical, Annie, to myself. Little did Chris know I was walking behind him, lip syncing one of my favorite show tunes, all while making grand gestures with my arms, just like Annie did. Chris never noticed my antics behind him, but I wish he had.

Chris could make me laugh until I couldn't breathe during some of the most challenging parts of our hikes. My tone-deaf singing voice and dramatic stage gestures likely would have unearthed a good chuckle from him. And he needed it after a poor night's sleep. My shyness in that moment became one of the few regrets I had during our entire FKT.

While we were making our final descent down Hyatt Ridge Trail, energized by my spectacular performance of "Tomorrow" that no one witnessed, I said to Chris, "I have a good idea for our daily photo. We should pretend we're finishing a marathon and string some of the flagging tape I keep in my backpack across the steel bridge. We can run through it while we set the timer on my phone to take a picture." Since a marathon is 26.1 miles, and we were wrapping up our twenty-sixth day, it felt fitting. I especially liked the irony of the shot—it would be the only time we'd actually ever run during our attempt. We had hiked every single mile so far, and it was important to us to say that we had *only* hiked, not run, the FKT.

It took more cajoling than usual to convince Chris to take the time to set up the more complicated photo. He needed sleep, and I'm sure he wondered how much rest he'd find in a home that included three teenagers. But by the time we reached the bottom of the trail and started setting it up, I knew he was all in. We ended the day on a high note, as we often did when we were the most tired, laughing at the first couple of failed attempts to time the photo properly with my phone. Afterwards, we headed towards Waynesville. As I made the last turn into my neighborhood, I got nervous. I knew my family missed me and we'd want to catch up, especially my kids who I hadn't seen in ten days, but I also knew how much Chris and I needed to rest after we ate dinner.

After big hugs from everyone and Josie passing gas right on cue, I could tell Larry had briefed the kids—reminding them we were still amid the FKT attempt and needed to stay focused and rested. They sat with us as we ate, and Paige braided my hair while Chris and I jumped on my Facebook page for a livestream, to update our friends and followers about our day.

A couple of days prior, I had made a post on my blog's Facebook page, announcing that we planned to finish at Baxter Creek Trail in the late afternoon of our twenty-eighth day of hiking, as long as Hazel Creek Trail stayed closed. As of that evening, there was nothing on the park's website showing it was open again or when they planned to reopen it. Our followers were eagerly expecting this announcement—many of them had already started nudging us to disclose our planned finish date, so they could arrange their schedules to celebrate with us at the finish. Time was running out, so we made the announcement with the caveat that it might change, depending on what happened with Hazel Creek.

The image of finishing, surrounded by people who supported us and loved us, was exactly how I wanted our story to end. But as with most things in life, it was out of my control. The only thing I could control was my reaction. I drifted off to sleep shortly after dinner, feeling optimistic that the trail would stay closed and we'd be able to finish the way we wanted.

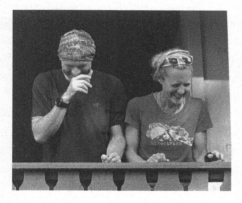

DAY 26: Slaphappy at the end of the day.

CHAPTER TWENTY-EIGHT

Bobcats of the Smokies

Oh my Lord, just look and see,
Smoky Mountain Mama took a hike with me.
Hair of gold and eyes of blue,
a cloud of dust and away she flew.

—DOUG PETERS, *I'M HER THORN, AND SHE'S MY ROSE*
(A SONG WRITTEN ABOUT OUR FKT)

Day 27—30.9 miles
(5099' gain, 6444' loss)

The sound of an angry cat cry filled the darkness of the cool morning air. And it sounded close. "What in the...that sounded like a cat," I said nervously, trying to calm my pounding heart, which was now beating fast from more than just exertion. In all my years practicing veterinary medicine, I had never heard a domestic cat make a sound like that, or as loudly—and I had treated my fair share of irate feral cats who wanted nothing to do with the humans trying to help them. Bobcats were naturally reclusive, so it would be highly unusual for one to make its presence known as we passed it in the dark.

Although mountain lions once roamed southern Appalachia, it was debatable whether any still lived in these woods. However, various trail cameras had supposedly caught a handful over the past few years, likely catamounts who had migrated from the west or pets that had escaped from their owners. It felt inconceivable that we were being stalked by an angry one, especially since we were such a large group, yet I couldn't think of another species of cat that could make that loud of a noise.

We were hiking on Cataloochee Divide Trail with my friend, Doug Peters, who asked if he could join us for a segment of one of our routes. Doug and I met several years prior at the Great Smoky Mountains Institute at Tremont, both taking courses to become certified naturalists. We were also fellow Experts in Residence at The Swag, a premier mountain inn bordering the park and Cataloochee Divide Trail. Doug, whose larger-than-life personality always entertained and amused, peppered us with questions about our endeavor as we hiked. Lane was also with us, and I treasured the time with both of my friends.

Doug, the last person hiking in our foursome, turned around after we heard the fierce feline cry. "Aaaahhh!" Doug yelled. I whipped around and saw his startled body leap violently backwards. For a moment, I couldn't tell what he had seen, but adrenaline coursed through my body in response to his frightened yell.

That's when I saw the 6-foot-tall cat that had scared Doug so badly. He was wearing a headlamp and hiking clothes. It was Bill Zimmerman, another friend and fellow search and rescue team member. He had planned on joining us that morning, but had overslept. Bill, a natural athlete, soon caught up with us on the trail. When he heard our voices in the distance, he couldn't resist the prank. "Oh my God, Bill, I should have known!" I exclaimed, howling with laughter.

Lighthearted antics and jokes were commonplace amongst our search and rescue team members. It often brought much-needed levity to otherwise sobering situations. Doug, however, was not used to such behaviors and did not start laughing with the rest of us. He was still processing the fact that he wasn't about to be taken down by a wild cat. Bill apologized quickly for startling him so badly.

Doug, who has a great sense of humor when he's not fearing for his own life, recovered after a few minutes. And Bill earned the trail name "Bobcat" that morning. Chris and I walked away with the biggest reward, though — belly aching laughter in the company of friends, even if it was at Doug's expense.

We parted ways with Doug, Lane, and Bill at The Swag, after I stopped by the guest reception desk and picked up my custom orthotic insoles that Larry had brought by for me. I had taken them out of my shoes to dry overnight, and I forgot to replace them in my sleepy stupor that morning. The risk of injury was always lurking in the shadows of our FKT, and the last thing I needed was a stress fracture this close to our finish.

Our time spent with friends that morning set the tone for the day, and we both felt as if we had an injection of energy as we made a double loop on several trails that emerged from Cataloochee Valley. It was less than forty-eight hours before our big finish and the weather was picture perfect with the bonus of lower humidity. And we were cruising along a network of trails that felt like a second home to me, given their proximity to Waynesville. My body was ready for the FKT to wrap up and my family was tugging at my heartstrings, but I was also sad that my long sojourn in this sacred place would soon end.

I had sought its solace and counsel during the major milestones of my entire adulthood—my engagement and eventual marriage; my pregnancies and the birth of two children, and the adoption of a third; and a time in my life when I needed its comfort the most — the loss of my mother. I came to these ancestral lands to celebrate my highest of highs and my lowest of lows. It seemed fitting to create another significant milestone within its boundaries, putting it center stage for a change.

As we traversed the ridgelines of the higher elevations where we had cell reception, I checked the park's website repeatedly for information about Hazel Creek. Nothing. The cause of the hiker's death still hadn't been released either, which wasn't unusual, but troubling all the same, since it didn't appear to have a simple answer.

Our route ended in the early evening on Rough Fork Trail, and we had to walk along the dirt road at the trailhead to our car, about a mile distant. Flooding had severely damaged the road months prior, and the park was still working on repairing it—everything was delayed because of the COVID-19 pandemic. Locals and tourists still flocked to it by foot though, eager to watch bull elk bugle in the meadows.

I was busy watching the elk when I heard Chris say, "Someone in that truck ahead just called out your name." I focused my attention on it and heard a voice call out again over the speaker on the truck's roof, "Hey Nancy!" It had to be someone from the park service since they blocked the road to visitors. As we approached the driver's side window, I peered in and saw my friend Brandon, one of the park's wildlife biologists, sitting in the passenger seat.

I had met Brandon the year prior during a search and rescue operation. One of The Swag's guests, Kevin Lynch, who suffered from early onset dementia, had wandered into the park by himself, unbeknownst to his family. It was a massive multi-agency search involving sixty agencies from five states. We found Mr. Lynch alive five days after he went missing. I was on the team that helped bring him down the mountain once he was found. Most 5-day searches in similar conditions didn't end this well. Tears of relief, surprise, and joy were shed that day, including some from SAR team members who had looked so tirelessly for Mr. Lynch in the dense and treacherous off-trail landscape of this area.

Brandon and I were on the same team searching for Mr. Lynch, and I instantly liked him. We kept in touch through social media after the search ended. He even met Aidan on Hazel Creek on the day the bear was euthanized in campsite 82.

"Hey Brandon, it's so good to see you!" I said excitedly. He and the ranger driving the truck were in the valley to monitor the elk-watching scene. It wasn't uncommon for park visitors to engage with the elk, attempting to feed them or take selfies with them. All the more reason to raise proper funding for the PSAR program, to educate visitors about proper etiquette and behavior around wildlife and save them from themselves sometimes, I thought to myself.

Knowing that Brandon would likely have some information about Hazel Creek, I didn't hold back asking him if he knew of the park's plans to reopen it or not. "Actually, we're heading to campsite 82 tomorrow to check the cameras again." He explained that the first time they checked the cameras, no bears had returned to the campsite. But the park kept it and the trail closed awhile longer, given the gravity of what occurred there. The following week, they went again, and a bear appeared in the footage. On this trip, however, they were given a directive. If the cameras didn't capture bear activity, the campsite would remain closed, but the trail would reopen.

"Are you serious? Tomorrow? We're supposed to finish this FKT the day after tomorrow, so that's really going to present a challenge for us." Chris replied. We were both frustrated at hearing this news, and it was hard to hide our reaction.

Brandon sensed our frustration and offered to message me as soon as he could with news of what they discovered. It was the best they could do, even if we didn't want to hear the news they might tell us. I was grateful for his consideration and waved as they drove away.

"I can't believe this is happening just as we're about to finish." I said, doing my best to keep my voice lowered in the company of the elk-loving tourists. And what were the odds of us running into the exact two rangers who would check the cameras at campsite 82 the next day? They were minuscule, but the challenge it potentially created for us felt as enormous as the park's acreage.

I wanted to be grateful to have the extra time to figure out what to do if the trail reopened. But now that we could see the finish line on the horizon after another long day on our feet, we were ready to cross it. Plus, it meant we'd need to hike twenty-one additional miles and add nearly an extra day to a record that otherwise would have stood solid at twenty-eight days.

Ever since discovering the moon cycle correlated to our attempt on the first night we started hiking, I looked for it each day. It became both my timekeeper and my fortune teller—its waning corresponding with my lowest moments on trail, and its waxing a symbol of my fullness as we neared the end. I'd knew I'd never look at it the same way again.

Ultimately, it was better that we knew. That way, we had some sort of timeline to base our alternate plans around. Now the challenge became figuring out how to best slay the dragon and get it done if need be.

Despite our frustration, we never lost sight of how trivial our situation was in the grand scheme. A hiker's death had brought us to this juncture. Our problem really wasn't a problem at all, just a challenge to fit some new pieces into the jigsaw puzzle. We spent many hours of our hikes speculating about all the ways the hiker could have died that weren't from a bear attack. It was the only way we could feel at peace for his untimely death.

That night, we inhaled our well-earned calories at my house and came up with two plans before heading to bed, each contingent on Hazel Creek and whether it reopened.

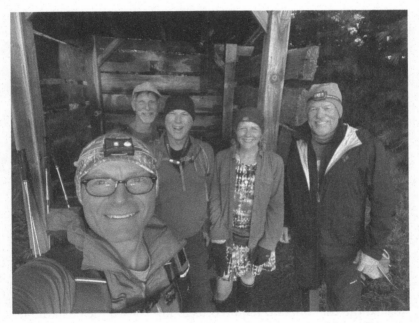

DAY 28: Chris, Bill Zimmerman, Lane DeCost, Nancy, and Doug Peters.

CHAPTER TWENTY-NINE

News from
the Back of Beyond

*"When you have exhausted all the possibilities,
remember this—you haven't."*

—THOMAS EDISON

Day 28—34.8 miles
(5939' gain, 6890' loss)

We started our long day in Cataloochee Valley on the Boogerman Trail, climbing steadily out of the valley before descending onto Caldwell Fork Trail with its many unbridged stream crossings. In one area, a natural event—probably a flash flood—had completely washed the trail out and required us to hike down the creek rather than above it.

We laughed as we slogged through the frigid water, remembering a winter hike when we did the same thing. Our feet felt like frozen blocks of ice by the end of the hike, and we dubbed them "Frankenstein Feet," since our gait resembled his. We always knew we were in for classic "Type 2" fun—the term hikers gave to trail conditions that caused distress but inspired entertaining stories to tell afterward. Normally, I reveled in the wild landscape of the Cataloochee area.

But with a nearly 35-mile day ahead of us, plus Hazel Creek Trail if it reopened, I was less enamored than usual.

We exited on Big Fork Ridge Trail and walked the same road as the night before, where we encountered Brandon and the other ranger. It felt like an eternity ago, given how much we packed into every hour. But one thing remained constant—we still didn't know Hazel Creek's fate.

We retrieved our extra pair of shoes and socks that Chris carefully hid in the woods, knowing our slog through Caldwell Fork would soak our original set. We left our wet shoes for Lane and Steve Kuni, friends from my SAR team, to retrieve for us when they moved my camper van to Deep Creek later that day. Our feet were well accustomed to staying wet by now, but we weren't fools if given the chance to keep them dry longer.

About a mile up Palmer Creek Trail, we came to a water crossing that Chris could rock hop. I could tell the last two rocks would be a stretch for me, but I hated to get my feet wet again with so much mileage left to cover. But it was safer to trudge through and get them wet—I would not risk an injury in the name of dry feet, even if I'd pay a price later when they hurt from maceration. Chris, ever the good friend, wasn't having it. Determined for me to keep my feet as dry as his, he picked up a fairly flat rock on the bank and set it in the water, so I'd have more stones to hop across before reaching the bank. He even stood waiting to catch my fall, in case the transitional rock he placed wasn't enough to prevent me from slipping.

This simple but kind act from Chris didn't surprise me. But as we continued on hiking, it stirred up emotions that had been brewing the last few days as we neared the end of our FKT journey together. "I know our friendship is unconventional, and some people think it's weird how much time we spend together out here. But we know there's nothing shady going on, and Jamie and Larry know they can trust us," I said to him, my voice cracking.

I took a deep breath and continued. "It's just that you're one of my best friends, and I hope you'll still want to hike together after all this FKT craziness." I felt better saying the words out loud, even if it led to discovering that Chris felt differently. Chris didn't seek hiking companions, and he often hiked solo before we teamed up. But his easygoing, friendly, and trustworthy manner made him a magnet for other hikers, and it wasn't surprising that people gravitated to his company on the Appalachian and Pacific Crest trails.

Chris reassured me that our friendship was important to him too and that I could call on him anytime I wanted to hike together. "Good! I'm glad that's settled, because I didn't want to have to stalk you," I said, laughing—all while keeping stride with his steady pace ahead of me as we climbed the mountain, just as we had done countless times before. Throughout the entire FKT, I expected the tension and stress of the endeavor to carry over into a quarrel between us at some point. But it never came to be, further validating how well we worked together as friends and teammates. Setting a speed record was important to me, but keeping our friendship intact was worth way more.

What was also still important to me was ending our FKT in the company of friends, family and our supporters, including Friends of the Smokies. This became increasingly clear to me after my emotional conversation with Chris, and I began revisiting the plans we hatched that were contingent on Hazel Creek reopening or not.

The night before, we came up with two plans. The first plan accommodated everyone who wanted to come to Big Creek on Friday, the day we had already announced we'd finish the FKT, assuming Hazel Creek remained closed. But we switched the order of our final two routes, to make car shuttling logistics easier if Hazel Creek opened and we had to hike it, too.

If Hazel Creek reopened, we'd only visit for a short while with whoever showed up at Big Creek. Then we'd drive to Clingmans Dome to hike Hazel Creek Trail and officially finish our FKT at the junction of Hazel Creek and Cold Springs Gap Trails in the dead of night, with no one there but the two of us. Nothing about that plan delighted me as I ruminated on the connections with the people I loved most in the world.

I proposed an alternative to Chris. If Hazel Creek reopened, we could head back to my house after we finished the route we were currently hiking. We would catch a quick nap before heading to Clingmans Dome to hike the Hazel Creek route. We'd return to my home, catch another brief nap, and then start our last route to end at Big Creek, just a day later. Chris liked the plan.

We knew our family and Friends of the Smokies could accommodate that change, and we'd just have to hope that most of our other supporters could still be there too. The only downside was that it would add more time to our FKT compared to the first alternate plan. With the new plan I devised, we'd retrace miles we'd hiked previously during our attempt. Unfortunately, no matter when we hiked it, we were still facing twenty-one extra miles under our feet. But we were willing to trade the time penalty to finish the attempt with our loved ones. Besides, despite the added time, we were still well on schedule to improve Jeff Woody's record by nearly four days. We would be the first people to hike all the trails in the Smokies in under thirty days.

At 4:25 that afternoon, I received a message from Brandon while we were hiking on Mount Sterling Ridge Trail—ironically near the same spot Chris and I first spoke about our individual plans to go after the FKT. "No bears on camera. So trails going to be open," his message read. We called Lane who confirmed that the backcountry office was telling people it was now open, too.

I was grateful to know our fate, but my stomach lurched at the thought of ending a nearly 36-mile day by tacking on another twenty-one miles in the dark of night—down a trail that hadn't been used in nearly a month. With two dozen unbridged creek crossings, the thought of walking up on unsuspecting bears at night didn't appeal, either. We were both frustrated that it reopened so close to our finish, but whining about it wouldn't solve anything. So we redirected our attention to setting the stage for success.

While we both had cell reception on the ridge, we called Jamie and Larry to share the news. Next, we knew we needed to get back across Fontana Lake once we finished hiking Hazel Creek. It would require hiking an additional six miles if we hiked all the way out to Fontana Dam. A boat shuttle would save hours of time and energy.

Ronnie, the private boat shuttle operator we used earlier, was out of town. Fontana Dam's marina only provided shuttles at designated times during the day, and if we missed the noon pick up time, it would be late afternoon before they returned. It was the only choice we had though, so we calculated the time it would take to hike twenty-one miles and gave ourselves a comfortable cushion in case we were running late.

The rest of that evening's route passed as slow as molasses. I knew that every minute we hiked was a minute I was losing to rest before our last push of the remaining fifty-two miles. We finished the route by hiking down Baxter Creek Trail, which was the trail we originally intended to end our FKT on. We thought it would be fun, and especially meaningful to Chris, to end the FKT on a trail with a name similar to Baxter State Park, where Mount Katahdin stood at the northern terminus of the Appalachian Trail.

As we crossed the bridge just before the trailhead, I imagined what the scene would be like if we had finished on this route as originally planned. But there was no time to dwell on these thoughts. We needed to hightail it to Waynesville and get some sleep.

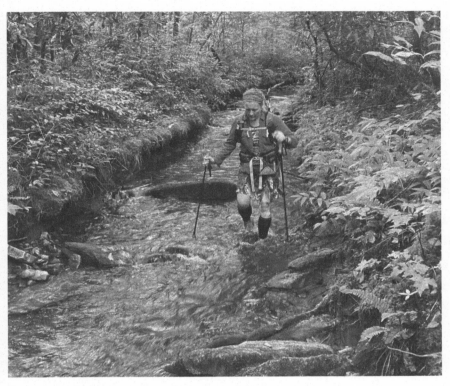

DAY 28: Slogging through Caldwell Fork Trail.

CHAPTER THIRTY

Leave Takings

Life contains inevitable partings and inescapable pain.
It is my belief that where there is love, relationships are unbreakable.
I could not bear letting go if I did not believe that.

—MARTHA MERCURE (MY MOM)

Day 29—52.1 miles
(5723' gain, 12,504' loss)

Similar to the first day of our FKT, my alarm sounded off at an unreasonable hour. I rose at 1:00 a.m. and felt as if I had just climbed
into my bed. I nearly had, considering only three hours had passed.
But twenty-eight days had also passed, and my voice wasn't cloaked
in doubt this time when I whispered to myself, "Here we go. Time
to set a record."

Larry had programmed the coffeemaker to brew a pot before we
left, and the familiar smell wafting into our bedroom when I opened
the door made life feel normal for just a moment. But there was
nothing normal about what we were leaving to do. For the first time
in the course of our FKT, I felt as if I was finally being forced to see
what my body could achieve.

Until that point, everything I had asked my body to do seemed like
a reasonable request. Over the course of the last twenty-eight days,

Chris and I discovered we'd underestimated how hard we could push ourselves, ending many days with unexpected reserves in our tanks (once I recovered from my injury). Now I would get the chance to see what the extra demand would feel like. It excited me as much as it scared me, digging deeper through our last miles when I was most fatigued from the cumulative effort.

We jumped in Chris' car and headed towards Clingmans Dome. We arrived at the parking lot, noting that the temperature gauge on the dashboard registered 35 degrees Fahrenheit outside. Powerful wind gusts pulled the car door out of my hand as I opened it, and I added more layers to my body to protect myself against both wind chill and air temperature. We ducked into the woods quickly, and the wind abated with tree cover.

The moon was one day past full, and it danced in and out of the scattered clouds. We barely needed an artificial light source on the high, exposed ridges to see the trail ahead of us. But when we passed the junction of the Appalachian Trail and Goshen Prong, the dark forest engulfed us and blotted out the moonlight.

As I always did at this junction, I reflected on Susan Clements and what I suspected might have been her fatal move by leaving the trail near this spot. I also remembered one of Elizabeth's videos and how she returned to this area two months after her mom died. She discovered flagging tape hanging on trees beside the trail with the date her mom went missing written on one of them. It was a revelation to Elizabeth, discovering search and rescue teams made it to this point the night her mom got lost, even though it was too late and Susan had already left the trail. "That made me feel so much better knowing they did go out there that night," she told her audience. And now—near the end—it felt especially poignant to be in the same spot since I'd made every step in Susan's memory. Perhaps there are no coincidences.

Soon after, we dropped off the Appalachian Trail and into inky shadows cast by Welch Ridge. After hiking nearly two more miles, we dropped onto Hazel Creek Trail—the trail that had interrupted our well-laid plans to complete our FKT in twenty-eight days. It commanded our full attention. The trail was badly eroded and off camber in many places, requiring careful foot placement and balance. At nearly thirteen miles, it was one of the longer trails in the park. The unbridged creek crossings made the first 8.7 miles the most challenging—many of them swift and thigh deep after recent rainfall.

Every time my foot slipped on the trail, I got angrier and more emotional, worrying that I'd injure myself and not be able to finish the FKT with Chris. "The irony of hiking a sketchy trail in the middle of the night while raising money for the park's preventive search and rescue program isn't lost on me," I seethed. "But here we are, hiking it when the park could have easily kept it closed one more day."

Of course, we were hiking the trail in these conditions under our own volition, and the park was rightfully indifferent to when we wanted the trail to reopen. I knew these facts, but my sleep-deprived emotional rant continued, anyway. It wove its way from irrational anger to pontificating on why two exceptional mothers, both mine and Susan Clements, had to die at much younger ages than their expected life spans.

Finally, I recognized my emotions for what they were stemming from—grief. I was on the cusp of achieving a goal that made me feel more alive than I'd felt in the ten years since my mom's death. Yet the tragic and premature death of someone else's mother had been the catalyst for the whole thing. My mother's death and its impact on me had brought me to the point of this achievement, too. Yet I would trade it all back in an instant, just to have her alive again. The juxtaposition of joy and grief, life and death—how it's all inextricably connected—became overwhelmingly apparent.

I began crying and couldn't stifle my sobs. Chris, who was likely wishing for a less-emotional friend to hike with since he was just as fatigued as I was, still took the time to be a good friend. He stopped hiking, turned around, and gave me a hug. "I'm sorry," I said through tears. "I'm so tired and I shouldn't be talking about this stuff right now." Saying the words aloud helped me regain my composure and refocus my attention on the task at hand.

The first light of day appeared towards the bottom of the trail, and I held back a short distance to pee. When I looked down at the ground, I noticed a dainty woodpecker feather in front of me, speckled with black and white polka dots. I had grown accustomed to hearing the call of a pileated woodpecker nearly every day of the FKT. The sound of persistence—drilling into the tough exterior of hardwoods—always reminded me of my mom's dogged determinedness to survive. I knew it wasn't a coincidence when I found the feather there. "I see you, Mama," I whispered to her softly.

Soon after the trail started leveling out from its long descent, we reached campsite 82. We found a note hanging from the wooden sign with the campsite number engraved on it. The note read, "Nancy East +1 The rest of your group is located at campsite #83 (approx. 2 miles). Please proceed to that site." It was a sobering reminder of the events that transpired, and it also revealed the answer to a question we had asked—if we had arrived at the junction of Welch Ridge and the Appalachian Trail earlier that fateful day, before the trail closure sign was placed, we could have legally hiked it.

We entered the campsite and quickly spotted two motion-activated trail cameras hanging in it, as well as a tent staged by the National Park Service, to see how bears might react to it. We looked across the creek to where Patrick Madura's body had been discovered by hikers. His cause of death was still a mystery at that time. No one was certain if he died from a bear attack or if the bear was simply taking advantage of an easy food source. And if that was the case, what caused his death? That they discovered him on the other side of the creek from the campsite only deepened the mystery. Passing this location and the area where Susan Clements got lost were blunt reminders of how trivial my annoyance was that Hazel Creek Trail reopened before we finished our FKT.

The remaining miles were the easiest on our bodies, but we were both feeling sluggish after covering forty-five miles in the last twenty-four hours. To distract ourselves from our fatigue, we hatched an idea for our twenty-ninth day photo. We reached the boat shuttle pickup point near Proctor with thirty minutes to spare and sat down for a much-needed break off our feet. But we didn't nap, at least initially. Instead, we set up the photo, highlighting our favorite junk food that we had eaten over the course of the FKT.

I represented the number nine, which required me to lie on my back to keep the food from falling off my face. I hung two broken Funyuns from my ears, placed a Haribo peach candy over one eye and a Brach's pumpkin candy over the other. For the remaining five numbers, I positioned five Mike and Ike candies across my teeth, doing my best to purse my lips around their edges to keep them in place.

Chris could say nothing about how ridiculous I looked, because it would send the candy flying if I laughed. Refraining from laughing became one of the biggest challenges I experienced during the FKT. It must have been equally agonizing for Chris to withhold his commentary. But he wanted the shot too, so he painstakingly kept his wit to himself. He quickly stuck two gummy worms up his nostrils to represent the number twenty and took a selfie of both of us lying on our backs facing the bright midday sun.

The photo sent us into a laughing fit when we looked at it on my phone's screen. Almost as quickly as we got riled up with humor, we sank into a sleepy spell against the warm rocks, taking advantage of every moment we had to rest, even when it only amounted to ten minutes.

The boat came and there was a big hiking group on it. They assumed we had camped the night before in one of the many campsites along Hazel Creek. "Oh, if they only knew," I thought to myself.

We boarded the boat and started our journey back across the lake, but not before I heard a hiker on the shore cry out, "Did one of you leave your hiking poles?" They were mine, and I was emotionally attached to them by now. I was still wearing a rigid splint on my left hand to keep my thumb immobile while my reattached thumb ligament healed. My poles were like an extension of my body, providing extra stability that wasn't there otherwise. I was certain they had kept me upright during many near slips in mud or on wet leaves and rocks, further protecting my ligament. I wasn't sure I would ever throw out a single piece of gear I used during our FKT attempt, especially my poles, and maybe even my splint, too. The boat driver returned so I could retrieve them, and we were back on our way.

I watched the Smokies as the distance between us grew, and it felt as if I had left an island on which they stood. Of course, they weren't on an island, but the landscape was indeed an oasis, surrounded by the impact of development and human civilization. What a treasure they were, majestically soaring high above it all.

Larry was waiting for us at the Fontana Marina with cold drinks packed in a cooler. A quick stop at McDonald's on the way back to our home, an hour and a half away, filled our bellies sufficiently before we took one more nap.

We rose in the early evening, ate dinner, filled two travel mugs to the brim with strong coffee, and set out for the last time. "I can't wait to see you at the end, and I love you so much. Thank you for trusting me and in my ability to do this," I said to Larry before we left, hugging him tightly.

While driving to the trailhead, I discovered a video message on my phone. It was from Jeff Woody. He delivered kind and supportive words, congratulating us in advance for our achievement. It was an impactful gesture, and I catalogued it in my mind, knowing that we too would have our record broken one day. Acting with humility and grace is where our own character would be put to the test.

We arrived at Mount Sterling Gap in the dark of the clear, cold night, snapped a quick photo at the trailhead to commemorate the occasion of our last route, and began hiking. The climb up Mount Sterling was easier than I expected. Similar to our first night of the FKT, I was jittery with anticipation and excitement. I wanted to soak in every minute of our last night, all too aware that I'd miss it once it was over.

At the Mount Sterling Ridge Trail junction, we turned around and began a quick descent. We turned onto Long Bunk Trail and bombed down it. It was in good shape for its infrequent use by hikers, and the gentle descent was a welcome change to our steep ascent of Mount Sterling. But even the most well-groomed trails have minor hazards that tired eyes might miss in the dark, poised to create problems for an unsuspecting hiker.

Such was the case for Chris when he tripped over a small root which sent his body flying in the air, headed straight for the sloped mountainside to the left of the trail. The terrain wasn't treacherously steep, but I watched his airborne body in horror until it contacted the earth again. Chris was face down and not moving. "Chris! Are you okay?" I screamed as I rushed towards him, terrified that he may have knocked himself unconscious or impaled his body on a fragmented snag. Chris was silent for a moment before he began peeling himself off the ground and back onto his feet. "I'm okay," he muttered. I had seen Chris fall many times before, but none of his previous falls incited such fear and alarm in me.

I nervously fired off questions and commentary in rapid succession. "Do you hurt anywhere? Do you need to rest? That was awful to watch and I can't imagine how it must've felt." Chris, wiping the dirt and debris off the front of his body, promised that he was okay and that we could carry on. I'm not sure who took longer to recover from the scare—Chris or me—but it validated the fact that the FKT wasn't ours until we took the very last step at the Big Creek trailhead the following morning.

After Chris' fall, we both needed a boost of laughter, the one trick in our bag that consistently worked to lift our spirits. So we worked hard at conjuring up our favorite memories of the last month. Perhaps it was too early though—the conversation felt forced. There would be time for celebrating and reminiscing, but not yet. We still had work to do.

We turned onto Little Cataloochee Trail, one of my favorite trails for its historical significance. A thriving community existed in this valley before the park's inception. Supporting evidence was in abundance along the trail. Two homes and the Baptist church, perched on a small knoll with an adjacent cemetery, were left intact and continue to be maintained by the park service.

In the small cemetery, the tombstones of infants were a stark reminder of the hardships in this bygone era and the thread of human grief that remains a constant across time and space. The inscription on Norma Palmer's monument, whose date of birth and death were the same, never ceased to give me pause—"A little bud of love. To bloom with God above. Our loved one."

We walked by the church, the nearly full moon now shining brightly overhead in the crisp fall air—natural and hand-crafted beauty coexisting in an environment born from Mother Nature. Unlike my mom and Susan Clements, she was unsympathetic to her creation, equipped with immutable power to blot out the very life that she gave, only to recycle and reuse the elements in perpetuity. Yet her grand design was the very thing that fed my soul. Ashes to ashes, dust to dust—perhaps even a speck of moondust exists within us all, I thought to myself.

The imposing scene of the church bathed in lumens and dancing in the shadows of the surrounding trees called to me. I stopped to capture it in a photo. "I need to remember this," I whispered to myself, while recognizing the impossibility of ever forgetting it. It failed to convey the emotions it evoked in the moment—but I'm not sure digital pixels are capable of such a thing.

We continued on through the night, mostly in silence, both fighting the heaviness of our eyelids, demanding more sleep. "I don't want it to end this way," I thought. Our camaraderie had taken center stage during our attempt, but neither of us had the energy to even speak to one another, much less draw from our tried-and-true conversation starters for a guaranteed chuckle.

Perhaps it was the way it was meant to end—sampling a taste of what our FKT could have been like had we tapped into our full physical potential. There was no way to know where our limits were, but it was clear to both of us we had not reached them, despite the challenges we endured along the way.

It was one of the greatest gifts of our journey. I had unnecessarily worried that I'd become unbearable to be with as the days wore on—the long and arduous miles limiting my ability to laugh and carry on meaningful conversations with Chris, focusing solely on finishing at all costs. But our FKT originated from human connection, both through our friendship and a desire to help others. Jeopardizing that in the name of a speed record would have been antithetical to our mission.

And maybe I had danced on the edges of my physical limits without even recognizing I was there. Undoubtedly, our companionship aided me each day, giving me a mental crutch to rest on when I needed it the most. While there was ample time to explore a dark cave of doubt and longstanding beliefs about my physical abilities, Chris was always there to set a line and help haul me out. Yet, I still had to cover the miles on my own. No one else could walk the trails for me.

Dawn arrived, bringing with it a lighter spirit and more energy from Chris and me. We made our way to Big Creek Trail, the last one on a long list, culminating in 948 miles of hiking. My mind swirled with an amalgamation of emotion, ranging from an eagerness to make our last step to never wanting it to end. I had hiked Big Creek Trail countless times with family and friends over the years—its treasures in every season were abundant.

But throughout the years, I'd brought less of myself with each return trip, pouring the bulk of my energy into tending to the needs of others. This wasn't a bad thing—it meant I had the good fortune of becoming a wife and mother, as well as a veterinarian. I wouldn't trade any of it, but the load grew heavier on my back through the years.

I rejoiced in the opportunity to do something for me and me alone. Hiking in the dead of night with the moon and stars guiding my way, I rediscovered what it means to set my personal bearing on the North Star and to follow it with all my might. Finishing successfully was always the goal, yet it held less weight than I expected at the end compared to the journey of arriving at this place.

We crossed the footbridge near the midway point on Big Creek Trail, and I looked down as Jamie had instructed us to do when we reached that point. A group of women who had supported us from afar every step of the FKT, including Kristen Mosley, our steadfast booster and bearer of trail magic as delectable baked goods, and Melissa Armour, whom we had met the day the Hazel Creek incident unfolded, had created the acronym "FKT" with small tree branches.

They had hiked the trail the prior day, planning to be at the trailhead when we arrived so they could congratulate us in person. When they couldn't rearrange their lives to return the following day, they left this love note for us instead. "Let's put our feet beside it and take a picture with them in it," I said to Chris, tears springing to my eyes, overwhelmed by the ongoing kindness of our many supporters.

We snapped the shot, treasuring what it represented—the last few miles of our long walk in the Smokies, culminating in the first time anyone would have ever hiked all her trails in less than thirty days. An arbitrary number, but one that mattered to both of us—and something I never thought possible within myself until I proved it so. As we started walking again, two trail runners whizzed by us in the opposite direction. I smiled widely while saying hello to them, unable to contain my excitement that the tortoises had indeed almost surpassed the hare.

The inherent tenet of an FKT attempt is one of speed—that one must be the fastest in order to succeed at achieving a record. But the path to achievement isn't always black and white. The ability to engage in relentless forward motion is a far more powerful attribute to possess—the great equalizer between athletes gifted with speed and the rest of us. We were not the first to prove this theory, but it was a crowning jewel to our success. What lives in the heart and mind are just as important, if not more so, than what manifests physically during an FKT.

As we approached the end of the trail, we started encountering people we knew—Kevin Fitzgerald, my friend and retired Deputy Superintendent of the park; Ramsey Roth, the primary record keeper for the Smokies 900 Challenge; and Benny Braden along with Sharon Spezia.

We walked with Kevin, Benny, and Sharon until we reached a point where we could see the trailhead in the distance, and they left us to join the crowd of people lined up on either side of the trail. I knew our families and Lane would be there, but I wasn't sure who else would give up their Saturday to make an appearance.

For the first time in the history of our friendship, I was speechless. It was impossible to summarize what we had endured together in just a couple of sentences, so I didn't even try. "I don't even know what to say right now. I'm just so proud of us," I said. "Me too," Chris replied as we stood there awkwardly, facing each other.

We gave each other a quick hug and reverted to the comfort of our familiar companionship. "Let's check each other's teeth and make sure there's no food hung up in them," Chris requested. We surveyed each other's gritted teeth while laughing, confirming that we were both in smile-worthy shape for photographs. "Okay, let's go finish this thing off before I get too emotional about it," I said excitedly, willing myself not to cry.

But I should have known better. As we drew closer, the gathered crowd held hiking poles in the shape of an overlapping arch over the trail, a symbolic rite of passage in the Smokies when someone finished the Smokies 900 Challenge, whether it was the first time or one of many. The simple gesture was all it took for the floodgates to open and my tears to flow. A few minutes after 10:00 a.m., we passed under the hiker tunnel twenty-nine days and ten hours after we started our FKT attempt. Sobs of joy and grief, love and loss, success and failure shook my body with a palpable awareness of how it's all intricately woven together in our humanity.

It reminded me of childbirth when the magnitude of my contractions became more than I could bear with my eyes open. I squeezed my eyes shut involuntarily, unable to open them even if I tried. Similarly, I couldn't look at the faces in the crowd without the need to close them and process the power of the moment internally. But now, instead of bringing another life into the world, I was redefining my own.

Chris side hugged me as we walked through the tunnel together. In his hug, I also felt the powerful embrace of the two women who had stood as sentinels by my side the entire time—my mom and Susan Clements.

My family was waiting at the end of the hiker tunnel, and I wept even more tears as I embraced them—those of gratitude. They were just as much a part of my success as I was, and it was only when I reached them that I felt the clock could officially stop on our success.

After gathering my composure, I turned to look back at all the people who joined us. My sisters and nephews were there, along with friends and people we knew from the Smokies hiking community. Even strangers who followed our journey online came to greet us.

Lane, of course, was there, too. I knew he was like a proud papa, watching us walk through the hiker tunnel. But we were just as proud of him for sticking with us through the entire endeavor, never wavering in his quest to get us to this point.

And finally, my eyes rested on more of my brothers from our search and rescue team. These men were more than just my friends and teammates—they were an extension of my family. I scanned the crowd, seeking each of them out in our orange team shirts they were wearing in solidarity.

Exposure to the razor-sharp edge between life and death creates an inherent bond among those who witness it together. Whether we were looking into the frightened eyes of a permanently injured person, walking someone out of the woods who was unscathed physically but not emotionally, or helping give a family an answer by bringing a deceased loved one's body back to them, our team was intimately familiar with unorthodox thin places. Perhaps the exposure to them is what gave us the fortitude to return, despite the emotional and physical risks of our job.

Mike Street, our team's leader, had organized a celebration down in the picnic area, complete with food and much-needed coffee. I was too excited to eat much, but I did my best to work the crowd and thank every single person in attendance.

Champagne was uncorked, and Tim Chandler, Executive Director of Friends of the Smokies, said a few congratulatory words. He also shared the news that we had raised $30,000 for the park's preventative search and rescue program. Chris followed with an eloquent speech and I fumbled through a heartfelt stream of sleep-deprived thoughts.

The crowd eventually cleared out. We packed up our belongings into our respective cars and said our goodbyes to Chris and Jamie. I felt a bit lost without a sense of urgency and intention to my actions, following the steady footsteps of my dear friend, "Pacer," into the healing mountain air. But I was also excited to head home and pack up for a beach trip on the South Carolina coast the following morning. Flat land would be a welcome change and the perfect place to reconnect with my family during our kids' fall break from school.

Larry backed our car out of the parking area, and we slowly drove past Chris and Jamie, who were packing up theirs. I glanced over at

Chris and smiled at him through the car window. His eyes met mine, and we exchanged a knowing glance. We'd poured every ounce of ourselves into a common goal that wouldn't have felt like a success unless we *both* made it to the end, side by side. We didn't need words in that moment to communicate our sentiment to each other. *Job well done, friend.*

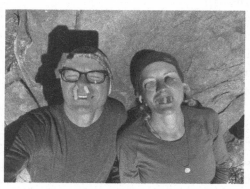

Waiting for the boat shuttle at Fontana Lake.

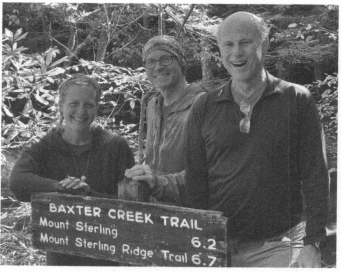

Nancy, Chris, and Lane at the beginning of the Benton MacKaye Trail on Day 29, where the first talks of attempting the FKT together began.

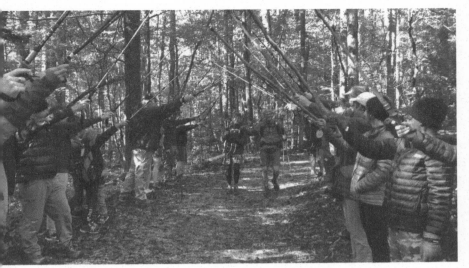

Family and friends salute at the finish at Big Creek Picnic Area.

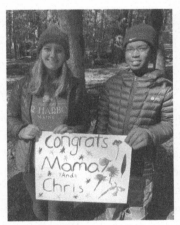

Paige and Wogene East.

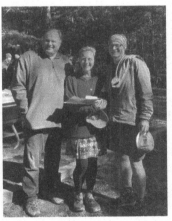

Friends of the Smokies Executive
Director Tim Chandler, Nancy, and Chris.

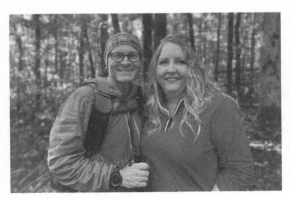

Chris and
Jamie Ford.

Epilogue

I came home from the FKT celebration and was determined to stay awake until evening so I could reset my sleep cycle. I lasted ten minutes before falling fast asleep, still in my hiking clothes. That evening, I unpacked my gear and food, only to turn around and repack my bags for our beach vacation.

Upon returning home from the beach, I fell back into my normal routines of parenting and life. But I longed for the trail and missed having an enormous goal to pursue. Post trail depression is a common occurrence among long distance hikers, but I didn't expect it to hit me as hard as it did. I was thankful to be back home and not have to adhere to a rigid schedule of training, but I still missed it.

Plus, I hadn't figured out what lessons I had learned from the experience and that bothered me. Only when I started writing this book a few months later is when the fog lifted and the lessons became clear. My hope is that they were obvious as you read through its chapters. Writing about the journey was also therapeutic for me. Bringing the story to life in words helped pull me out of my emotional slump.

My thumb continued to heal, but it was never the same. Despite months of hand therapy, scar tissue had formed around the central joint of my thumb. I did not regain full flexion of it, but it was enough to get by. My thigh recovered without any lasting consequences, but my hormones had a more challenging time. I felt as if I had been catapulted into perimenopause when hot flashes became a common occurrence following the FKT.

Chris and I were invited to attend a ribbon cutting ceremony for Trillium Gap Trail's reopening after its long restoration project. There, we learned that the money we raised helped Friends of the Smokies purchase supplies and equipment for the burgeoning PSAR program.

I continued to meet up for regular, arduous hikes with Chris. Even without a goal, we both craved endurance style hiking. And we loved recounting our many experiences together on trail as we hiked along, while creating new memories in the process. He remained (and will always be) one of my dearest friends.

My search and rescue team stayed busy as novice hikers continued to hit the trails in unprecedented numbers. Within eight months of finishing the FKT, we would be involved in the recovery of two male hikers, both deceased from fatal falls. One of them, Dustin Williams, was an acquaintance. My team recovered Dustin's body in dangerous terrain, our skilled rope technicians leading the effort. I knew how vulnerable my teammates were as they brought Dustin off the mountain, and I found myself in a unique position of mourning the loss of someone I knew while fearing for the well being of people I loved. That night, I vowed to further my training in order to be of more use in similar situations, namely by gaining more medical expertise with a Wilderness First Responder certification (which I completed a few months later).

I retired from my career in veterinary medicine to pursue a new path in guiding hikes and backpacking trips as well as writing. Before the FKT, I harbored guilt about leaving a career I had worked so hard to achieve, even though my heart was no longer in it. My long walk in the Smokies guided me down a path I didn't have the courage to take prior to that. I've never looked back from my decision.

On August 19, 2021, Great Smoky Mountains National Park issued a news release. It stated that the North Carolina Chief Medical Examiner released a final report confirming that Patrick Madura (the backpacker at campsite 82) likely died from trauma caused by a bear. The news was a sobering reminder that our public lands are wild spaces with inherent risks, no matter how prepared one might be.

What to Bring on a Hike

No matter how short your hike, I encourage you to *always* pack the "Ten Essentials." The Ten Essentials were originally assembled in the 1930s by The Mountaineers, a Seattle-based organization for outdoor adventurers, to prepare them for emergency situations in the out-of-doors. Now, the list has evolved to a "systems" approach. At first glance, it may seem excessive, but collectively these items do not add up to much weight and will easily fit into a small backpack.

❶ Navigation Map, compass (and knowledge of how to use them together). Hiking apps such as Gaia GPS (my preference) are excellent tools for navigation, but they shouldn't be your only method since technology can fail. GPS units are nice to have, but phone navigation apps are typically easier to use and usually have more robust features.

❷ Illumination Headlamp and/or small flashlight. Extra batteries or a portable battery charger are also recommended.

❸ First Aid A first aid kit should be tailored to your needs. Mine always includes a small supply of ibuprofen and diphenhydramine

(Benadryl) along with a small kit of bandaging materials and foot care for potential blisters or hot spots.

4 **Gear Repair** This should also be customized to your potential needs. My repair kit includes a small supply of duct tape (wrapped around a hiking pole), dental floss with an embroidery needle, and super glue. A small pocketknife is also included in my repair kit.

5 **Fire** Waterproof matches, a lighter, tinder, +/- a small back-packing stove. Also, make sure you know methods to build a fire, especially with wet wood.

6 **Shelter** This can be as simple as a trash compactor bag that also doubles as a liner for your backpack. If used as an emergency shelter, a small slit can be cut in the side of the bag, to be used for ventilation and breathing. I also carry a small emergency bivy that only weighs a few ounces. A lightweight, small tarp is also a great addition, and many weigh less than 8 ounces (I carry one made by Gossamer Gear).

7 **Extra Food** Bring slightly more food than you think you'll need, just in case you're in the woods longer than expected.

8 **Extra Water** Bring an ample supply of water for the route you're hiking, but also have a plan for purifying additional water, should you need it. I carry a Sawyer Squeeze Water Filter for this purpose, but there are many options on the market to consider.

9 **Extra Clothing** The type and amount of clothing varies, depending on where and when you're hiking. Also, make sure to carry rain protection at all times, even if there isn't rain in the forecast on the day of your hike. Bright clothing will usually help SAR teams locate you more quickly.

10 **Sun Protection** Sunglasses, sunscreen, and or protective clothing from the sun should be considered. I am a huge fan of Gossamer

Gear's Liteflex Umbrella for sun (and rain) protection. It also deters insects from hovering around my head.

*Optional but highly recommended A personal locator beacon such as a Garmin InReach Mini (what I carry) or ACR ResQLink. If you are using your phone for photography or navigation, a portable battery charger is recommended. A loud whistle is also highly recommended.

What to Do Before Leaving on a Hike

In addition to what you carry with you in your backpack on a hike, make sure to do the following before leaving home:

1 Leave an itinerary with someone and the estimated time you think you'll emerge from the woods. Check in with this person after you get off the trail.

2 Check the weather forecast for the day of your hike and a day or two further out.

3 Research the area you'll be hiking in before you set out. It's best to know elevation gain and loss, potential unbridged stream crossings, reliable water sources, etc. before you hit the trail versus when you're in the middle of a hike.

4 Pack as if you'll spend a night out in the woods waiting for a SAR team to come to your aid. As long as you have the "Ten Essentials System," you should be in good shape, but tailor what you bring according to the season and the weather forecast.

5 Put your phone in airplane mode or turn it off completely, to avoid draining the battery while you hike in areas without cell reception.

Final Notes from Nancy

One final item to pack doesn't cost or weigh a thing: *a positive mental attitude* (PMA). Should you become lost or injured, PMA is just as important as any gear you're carrying. I have consistently observed more favorable outcomes for our subjects who remain calm and optimistic about their outcome during their predicament.

The acronym STOP is also helpful, especially if you're lost. It stands for Stop, Think, Observe, and Plan. Stopping to think and act on logic rather than emotion, after observing your environment and what you need to do to stay alive in it, is a good way to plan during a stressful situation.

Remaining stationary if you're lost, especially if you're on a trail, will allow SAR teams to come to your aid much more quickly than if you are a moving target wandering through the woods.

If you'd like to stay updated on my speaking schedule or obtain more extensive information on hiker safety and preparedness, visit my website at *nancyeast.com*. I'd be honored to hear from you. Happy trails!

Sponsors of our
Hiker Safety Fundraiser

American Backcountry
*Appalachian Gear Company
Big Pig Outdoors
*BioLite
Bob Carr Photography
Boundary Life Gear
ESEE Knives
*Gaia GPS
*Gossamer Gear
*Injinji Socks
*Lightheart Gear
Kirby Phillips Artwork
Kristi Parsons Photography
*Paleo Valley
Plaasabilities Photography (Kristina Plaas)
*Point6 Socks
*Sawyer
The Swag
Up 'N Adam Adventures

* *Brands that Nancy and Chris used during the FKT. More specifically, we both used Gossamer Gear Kumo Backpacks and Nancy's beautiful hiking dresses were made by Lightheart Gear.*

Acknowledgments

This story was inspired by and stemmed from the love and loss of two irreplaceable mothers. I appreciate the time Susan Clements' family spent with me on the 10-year anniversary of my mom's death, when I asked for their blessing to weave Sue's tragic story into our FKT fundraiser and awareness campaign.

I am indebted to my editor, Steve Kemp, who was willing to take on this project and make it shine. I chose you because I knew your editorial expertise is top notch. But more than anything else, I treasured working with someone who loves Great Smoky Mountains National Park as much as I do. Your counsel and encouragement gave me confidence to publish this book. I started the project with an editor, but I ended it with a new friend.

Lisa Horstman, when I learned that you were the book's graphic designer, I was even more excited to publish it. I've long admired your talents and knew the project was in the perfect hands. Thank you for treating it with such care. It was instantly apparent how dedicated you are about creating something special for authors.

Gay Bryant, your loving heart created a masterpiece for the book's cover. I am forever grateful for your help on such a tight timeline.

Our fundraiser wouldn't have been nearly as successful without the support of many companies who contributed by way of donated products and services we auctioned off. These are companies I am proud to support with my own dollars, because they care about hiker safety and preparedness. They are listed on page 173, and I hope you will consider giving them your business, too.

Chris and I approached Friends of the Smokies with our wild idea, and it was Anna Zanetti's forward thinking that led it to fruition. Marielle DeJong, Sarah Herron, Julie Dodd, and Tim Chandler also played big roles in bringing the fundraiser to life. The park benefits immensely from the love and care you all pour into your jobs.

My countless friends and the hiking community who supported our effort were the wind at my back. Whether it was through donations, texts, replies on social media posts, trail magic in the form of homemade goodies or a shuttle ride, moving our cars around the park, offering us a place to sleep, hiking with us (even if it did take a few years off your life, Doug), chaperoning two teenage boys to Hazel Creek (with much more than you bargained for, Dawson), or simply thinking of us from afar, you pushed me forward each day.

To the special group of people who came to celebrate with us at the end of the FKT (and those of you who were with us in spirit because you couldn't be there in person), it was the best trail magic ever. I'll never forget any of your hugs or congratulatory words.

Kevin Fitzgerald, you are a class act in every way. My gratitude for your support, training advice, and encouragement before, during, and after the FKT is immense. That you believed in my amateur athletic ability to pull this thing off gave me more strength than you can ever imagine.

Matt Kirk, your humble athletic prowess and willingness to lend your counsel in the planning and training stages of our endeavor, motivated and inspired me. It was a blast watching your postman project unfold simultaneously, and I'm so thankful our paths crossed.

Heather "Anish" Anderson, your words had a huge impact on my life and planted the seed to attempt something I feared I couldn't achieve. Thank you for your guidance in the beginning stages of this manuscript. But more importantly, thank you for being a bright, shining light in the world.

Peter Bakwin, Buzz Burrell, and Jeff Schuler, the founders of the Fastest Known Time website, thank you for dedicating so much of your free time and energy to the platform and to the athletes it serves, even amateur ones like me. Seeing my name on the Smokies 900 page of the website still gives me chills.

A special thanks to Eric Yarrington of Yarrington Physical Therapy. Your devotion to our community's health is readily apparent, and your expertise is always trustworthy and helpful. A heartfelt thanks for your time and loving care on a Friday night, when I feared the worst about my injury.

Dr. Doug Gates, thank you for your skilled hands and for trusting that I'd protect your good work during the FKT. Kelsea Sonnier, I never thought I'd say I looked forward to attending my many hand therapy sessions, but your friendly demeanor and our shared interests made it so.

I stand in awe of the dedication of Great Smoky Mountains National Park Rangers, protecting and preserving our public lands. I know your jobs must often feel thankless, but know my appreciation is infinite. Rangers Will Butler, Brandon Garcia, Matthew River, and Rene' Williams, a special thanks for your support and friendship.

Jamie, I can think of few people as selfless as you. I carried your trust, dedication, and love with me every step of the way. Chris may have your heart, but I appreciate you sharing it with me, too.

To my brothers and sisters of Haywood County Search and Rescue, I walk with my heroes during our operations. Your unwavering dedication to serve others, no matter the risk to yourself, inspires and pushes me to challenge myself in the same way...so that others may live.

Lane, stand by because I know a guy! Chris and I had the easy part of the job hiking the routes compared to creating them and their corresponding spreadsheets. Your tireless work in the hiking community to keep people "safe and found" is to be commended, also. I hope you know how much you mean to me, friend.

Amanda, Molly, Daniel and Chad, thank you for helping Larry hold down the fort in my absence. Jennifer and Daddy, caring for the kids on short notice so Larry could join us for a few days was an unexpected treat when I needed it the most. To the rest of my family, your words of encouragement from afar were always with me, too. A special thanks to Isaac for your sherpa services and staying calm during an unsettling backpacking trip.

To Chris, my partner in all things that defy rational thinking, this story is colorful and lively because of our friendship. I still can't believe you agreed to attempting the FKT together, and I still pinch myself that we pulled it off. Here's to many more miles and memories, especially if they involve Funyuns and bear costumes.

To Aidan, Paige, and Wogene, of all my various roles and titles, "Mama/Mom" is the most sacred to me. Thank you for giving me your blessing to fulfill a dream and feel as young as you are again. I carried all three of you in my heart every step of the way. As Paige used to say, "I love you all da time."

Larry, you are the yin to my yang and my unwavering rock. Your trust in my abilities and my character are what made this endeavor feel easy when nothing else did. Thank you for signing on to be a single parent while I was away and for every encouraging word and touch throughout the journey. It all helped fuel my beating heart up and down the mountains. I love you, always.

Ever since I was a little girl devouring Laura Ingalls Wilder's Little House books, I've dreamt of living an adventurous tale that's worthy of sharing with the world through my words. I hope this book inspires a grand adventure in your own life. Thank you for reading it.

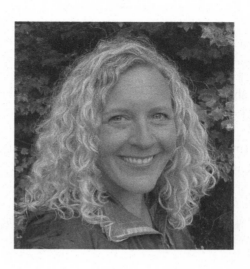

About the Author

Nancy East, an avid hiker and backpacker, is a firm believer that you're never too old to be what you might have been. After a 23-year career as a small animal veterinarian, she retired to pursue her passion as a writer, hiking guide, and speaker.

She is a member of Haywood County's Search and Rescue Team, a founding board member of the WNC Wilderness Safety Fund, a Gossamer Gear Ambassador, and a Southern Appalachian Naturalist. Nothing brings her more joy professionally than educating her fellow hikers about how to stay "safe and found."

In 2019, she and her good friend, Chris Ford, set the fastest known time (FKT) for a mixed-gender team on the Tour de LeConte Challenge. In 2020, they set the overall FKT for the Smokies 900 Challenge. Nancy has hiked all the trails in Great Smoky Mountains National Park four times, and she continues going back for more.

When she's not on the trail, Nancy is a mother to three children and a wife to her high school sweetheart. They live with their beloved dog in the mountains of Western North Carolina.

Visit Nancy at nancyeast.com.